Preface

The sections of this book are not placed in any particular order, and any part can be read without the necessity of reading an earlier section. It is intended as a collection of useful facts on a variety of subjects. The absorption, or secretion, metabolism, function, and excretion of substances are listed alphabetically in the first section. Details of various substances in this first section may be found to be useful in the second section, in which problems of over/underhydration with hypo/hypernatraemia, plus hypo/hyper-osmolality, are dealt with: e.g. sodium, osmolality, water, urea, plasma oncotic pressure, etc.

There is an analysis of metabolic/respiratory acidosis/alkalosis and combined disorder patterns in the third section, and reference to individual substances in the first section may again be useful, e.g. bicarbonate, hydrogen ion, potassium, etc. Since renal function is fundamental to homeostasis, a detailed account of renal structure, blood supply and detailed function is given in the fourth section, with reference to acid–base and water balance. The use of diuretics is universal, and therefore the mode, site of action and strength of action of different commonly used diuretics are described.

The fifth section describes various clinical problems (e.g. cardiac failure), demonstrating the fact that patients suffer from combined abnormalities, e.g. metabolic acidosis with renal failure plus over-hydration.

Finally, formulae are listed for simple calculation of deficit/excess, as guides during treatment, with a table of contents of commonly used readily available prepacked fluids.

Throughout the text [R] is placed against certain conditions, when only a few cases have been reported. When the inheritance of a disease or deficiency state is known this is shown as autosomal dominant [AD] or autosomal recessive [AR].

R. D. E.

Contents

How to use this book

Section 1
This largest section of the book contains information about absorption, function, regulation of concentration and excretion, of cations, including sodium, potassium, magnesium, calcium, and anions, including bicarbonate, chloride and phosphate, plus causes and effects of increased or decreased concentration. Metabolism and excretion of various organic substances, including urea, lactic acid and creatinine, are also described. Water and various body fluid compartments, including interstitial fluid and cerebrospinal fluid, are similarly described. Details of relevant hormones, including antidiuretic hormone, aldosterone, parathyroid hormone and renin, are given, again with causes of abnormal deficiency or excess. Included in the sections dealing with buffers, bicarbonate and carbon dioxide are sections describing the effects of clinical variations in plasma pK on calculated plasma bicarbonate, and the inter-relationship between P_{CO_2} and P_{O_2} (with particular reference to the respiratory drive in metabolic alkalosis). This section is intended for ready and rapid reference to information about individual substances, body fluids or laboratory measurements, such as plasma anion gap, base excess, etc.

Section 2
After a description of causes, signs and symptoms of hypovolaemia/hypervolaemia, hyponatraemia/hypernatraemia and hyperosmolar states, there are descriptions of causes, signs and symptoms, laboratory findings, physiopathology, and treatment of the various combinations of dehydration/normal hydration/overhydration with hyponatraemia/normonatraemia/hypernatraemia, arranged in a matrix about the normal state. In particular, the section dealing with overhydration and hypotonicity is expanded to include a detailed examination of the syndrome of inappropriate ADH release (SIADH).
Each individual section, e.g. dehydration and hyponatraemia, includes a description of causes, signs and symptoms, laboratory findings, physiopathology and treatment, where relevant.
References to details of individual substances, fluid compartments, etc. in Section 1, e.g. plasma sodium, interstitial fluid, bicarbonate, water, urea, osmolality, etc., and to sections in Section 3 (e.g. metabolic

alkalosis, or acidosis complication dehydration) may be helpful. Descriptions of diuretic therapy in Section 4 may also be useful.

Section 3
This section deals with metabolic/respiratory acidosis/alkalosis, and includes a description of signs and symptoms, causes and treatment of these various clinical conditions. Again, reference to descriptions of plasma hydrogen ion concentration (pH), $P\text{CO}_2$, respiration, chloride, ammonia in blood and ammonium excretion in the urine in Section 1, plus reference to Section 2 (e.g. metabolic acidosis complicated by severe dehydration), may be of help.

Section 4
Since the kidneys are responsible for continuous maintenance of homeostasis, with very rapid and continuous adjustments of plasma pH and $Pa\text{CO}_2$ via variations in the depth and rate of respiration, the structure and functions of the kidney are briefly described. This description is followed by details of the pharmacology of commonly used diuretics, with the rates of excretion of water, sodium, potassium, chloride and bicarbonate, where relevant. The clinical uses of the various diuretics are described, with their advantages and disadvantages, plus their toxic side-effects. Finally, there is a brief statement of the general complications of diuretic therapy—a therapy which consists either of overloading the kidney filtration and reabsorption system, or the deliberate poisoning of specific renal tubular enzyme systems.

Details in this section are relevant in the various sections describing treatment of clinical states in Sections 2 and 3.

Section 5
Various complex clinical syndromes, including cardiac failure and cerebral oedema, are described, in which the various syndromes described in Sections 2 and 3 may be compounded. Thus syndromes of dehydration/normal hydration/overhydration, and hypotonicity/normal tonicity/hypertonicity, are complicated by abnormal changes in hydrogen ion concentration, with, in addition, renal failure.

There is a simple brief table of contents of common fluids available for infusion, followed by simple formulae for calculation of excess, fluid, sodium deficit, etc. which may be useful in the planning of treatment.

The five sections are therefore meant to be used for rapid cross-reference in clinical practice. Greater detail on individual topics can be obtained from the large standard textbooks.

Abbreviations

ACTH	Adrenocorticotrophic hormone
ADH	Antidiuretic hormone
cAMP	Cyclic adenosine monophosphate
ATP	Adenosine triphosphate
AVP	8-Arginine vasopressin, antidiuretic hormone
CPK	Creatine phosphokinase
CSF	Cerebrospinal fluid
CT	Calcitonin
CVP	Central venous pressure
DDAVP	Vasopressin analogue
2,3-DPG	2,3-Diphosphoglycerate
EAV	Effective arterial volume
ECF	Extracellular fluid
ECG	Electrocardiograph
ECV	Effective circulatory volume
FFA	Free fatty acids
GFR	Glomerular filtration rate
ICF	Intracellular fluid
iCT	Immunoreactive calcitonin
iPTH	Immunoreactive parathyroid hormone
ISF	Interstitial fluid
NAD^+ (NADH)	Coenzyme I, nicotinamide adenine dinucleotide
$NADP^+$ (NADPH)	Coenzyme II, nicotinamide adenine dinucleotide phosphate
pH	$-\log_{10} C_H$, where C_H = hydrogen ion concentration
pK	$-\log_{10} K$, where K is the dissociation constant of a weak acid (or weak base)
P_{CO_2}	Partial pressure of carbon dioxide
Pa_{CO_2}	Partial pressure of carbon dioxide in arterial blood
P_{O_2}	Partial pressure of oxygen
Pa_{O_2}	Partial pressure of oxygen in arterial blood
PRA	Plasma renin activity
PTH	Parathyroid hormone
RNA	Ribonucleic acid
RPF	Renal plasma flow
SIADH	Syndrome of inappropriate antidiuretic hormone
T_4	Thyroxine

1. Individual Substances and Measurements

The absorption, or secretion, metabolism and excretion of substances are listed alphabetically, with estimations (e.g. osmolality) and their significance. These sections are useful when the subsequent sections are used.

Albumin
Aldosterone
Blood ammonia
Urine ammonium
Angiotensin II
Anion gap
Antidiuretic hormone (ADH)
Base excess/deficit
Bicarbonate
Blood–brain barrier
Buffers
Calcitonin
Calcium
Carbon dioxide
$Paco_2/Pao_2$ (partial pressures of carbon dioxide and oxygen in blood)
Cerebrospinal fluid
Chloride
Cortisol
Creatinine
Glucose

Hydrogen ion/pH
Interstitial fluid (ISF)
Lactic acidosis
Magnesium
Oncotic pressure/colloid osmotic pressure
Osmolality
Blood oxygen (Pao_2)
Paediatric problems
Parathyroid hormone (PTH)
Phosphate
Potassium
Renin
Control of respiration
Sodium
Thirst
Trace elements
Urea
Vitamin D
Effective arterial volume (effective circulating volume)
Water

ALBUMIN

Albumin is the main plasma protein, with a molecular weight of 66 300–69 000, and a circulating half-life of about 18 days in normal subjects. It has a relatively low intrinsic viscosity, a strong internal structure, and is heterogenous. With an iso-electric point between pH 5·4 and 4·4, it contains 584 amino acid residues, with an abundance of aspartic and glutamic acid residues, but only very small amounts of tryptophan.

It is synthesized in the liver, which produces up to 100 g of plasma proteins each day. In the liver cells, albumin is synthesized by free polysomes for use inside the cell, and by endoplasmic reticulum-bound polyribosomes for systemic release from the liver.

1

The concentration of tryptophan and certain other amino acids can 'turn on' albumin synthesis, and these are the same amino acids which 'turn on' urea synthesis. Albumin synthesis is increased by
1 Thyroid hormones.
2 Insulin.
3 Human growth hormone.
4 Testosterone.
5 ACTH.
6 Adrenocortical hormones.

Albumin can bind reversibly with both cations and anions. Protein-bound calcium fraction is bound, 90 per cent to albumin and 10 per cent to globulin, in the plasma. The calcium ions are bound to the albumin molecule by chelation to a pair of adjacent carboxyl groups on glutamyl or aspartyl residues, and there are 12 independent binding sites per albumin molecule. This is very relevant in the assessment of hypocalcaemia in the presence of hypoalbuminaemia.

Albumin also carries bilirubin, a small proportion of thyroxine (T_4), and many drugs after their ingestion.

The normal adult has 4–5 g/kg body weight of exchangeable albumin, one-third of which is intravascular. Half of the total plasma albumin escapes from the capillaries every day, to be returned to the blood stream via the lymphatics; 10–20 g (6–10 per cent) are degraded each day.

Eighty per cent of the oncotic action (colloid pressure) of plasma is due to albumin. It is thought that changes in the oncotic pressure at or near the sites of synthesis control the rate of albumin synthesis. Following an infusion of a colloid, there is decreased synthesis of albumin, and following infusion of albumin resulting in colloid pressure above normal, there is suppression of albumin synthesis and also increased rate of degradation of circulating albumin.

Albumin can enter the peritoneal cavity
1 Directly through the liver capsule (probably the principal route).
2 From the plasma.
3 Via lymphatics communicating with the peritoneum.

In acute water overload, the skin can contain 37 per cent of the excess water, with some albumin; e.g. a 70-kg man with a volume excess of 5 litres of water absorbs excess water in his skin, the increased turgor of the skin only increasing by 1 mm.

Pathological

1. *Increase*

There is no pathological condition associated with abnormal excess of albumin, although this could arise as a result of iatrogenic misjudgement.

2. Decrease

   a Decreased synthesis.

   b Increased loss and degradation. Two examples of excessive loss:

      i Burns—massive shift of water and electrolytes into a sequestered site in cells during the first 24 hours after burning, with protein loss into the tissues, and from the denuded areas, because of marked increase in vascular permeability. There is also long-term depression of albumin synthesis which can last up to 60 days.

      ii Thoracic duct fistula—can lose 50 per cent of the daily production of albumin.

Therapeutic Use of Albumin Solution

1 Shock.
2 Burns.
3 Adult respiratory distress syndrome.
4 Occasionally

   a Acute liver failure.

   b Ascites.

   c Post-surgery with low plasma albumin, and poor healing.

   d Acute nephrosis.

Unjustified Use

To replace the daily synthesis of albumin (14–23 g per day).

ALDOSTERONE

Synthesis

Aldosterone is synthesized in the zona glomerulosa of the adrenal cortex. Plasma levels of aldosterone fluctuate between 5 and 20 ng/100 ml varying with the time of day, diet, etc. (i.e. 'squirter'). ACTH, angiotensin and potassium are necessary for aldosterone secretion to occur, secretion being ineffective in the presence of hypokalaemia. The macula densa detects stretch in afferent arterioles, and also detects changes in sodium concentration (osmolar) in arteriolar plasma and distal renal tubules.

   Angiotensin III acts on zona glomerulosa cells, with potassium entering the cells before aldosterone release. An increase in potassium concentration around the zona glomerulosa results in aldosterone release. After administration of potassium, renin activity is suppressed.

If ACTH is given by continuous infusion, corticosterone release is parallel to aldosterone release for 12–18 h. Peak production of aldosterone occurs at 36–48 h, is maintained for 24 h and falls away again, even though the ACTH infusion is continued. After a single dose or ACTH, aldosterone release is briefly stimulated, but its action is not sustained.

If a high concentration of salt reaches the macula densa, the macula densa cells take up sodium, where it is transported to renin-producing cells with which they are in contact. Renin enters the wall of afferent arterioles. Angiotensin precursor and converting enzyme in the arteriolar wall produce angiotensin II locally, causing arteriolar vasoconstriction, and hence reduction in the glomerular filtration rate.

Aldosterone Release

1 Erect posture for 3–4 h.
2 Diuretics.
3 Reduced ECF.

Synthesis

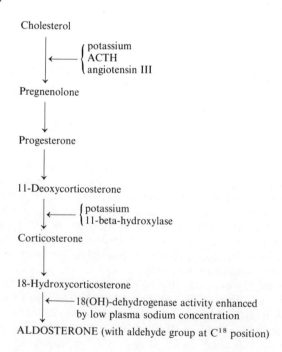

Cholesterol

← { potassium
    ACTH
    angiotensin III

Pregnenolone

Progesterone

11-Deoxycorticosterone

← { potassium
    11-beta-hydroxylase

Corticosterone

18-Hydroxycorticosterone

← 18(OH)-dehydrogenase activity enhanced by low plasma sodium concentration

ALDOSTERONE (with aldehyde group at C^{18} position)

Release

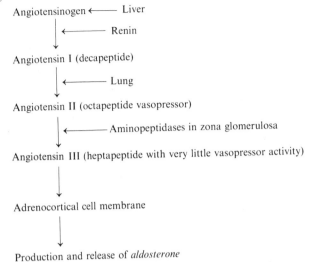

4   Sodium depletion.
5   Volume depletion.
6   Hypoperfusion of the juxtaglomerular apparatus (? reduction in salt passing the cells of the macula densa causing release of renin).

Aldosterone Action

Aldosterone acts on:
1   Proximal renal tubule cells.
2   Distal renal tubule cells.
3   Intestines.
4   Sweat glands.
5   Salivary glands.
(i.e. where sodium/potassium exchange occurs). In the kidney after synthesis of new proteins at the cell membrane and tubular lumen junction, as a result of RNA translocation with change in cell cytoplasm, transport of sodium across the distal tubule cell wall occurs, following synthesis of ATPase for sodium/potassium exchange. The peritubular cell membrane is acted on so that

     a   There is increased sodium reabsorption with passive potassium diffusion into the tubular lumen.
     b   Increased potassium concentration in the peritubular cells results in increased diffusion of potassium into the lumen.
     c   Increased permeability of tubular luminal cell membranes to both sodium and potassium develops.

Aldosterone Catabolism and Excretion

Its biological half-life is 30 min. Eighty to ninety per cent of the released aldosterone is inactivated at its first passage through the liver. It is converted to tetrahydroaldosterone, then conjugated with glucuronic acid, before excretion in the urine; 10 per cent of the released aldosterone is catabolized in the kidney to an 18-oxo-conjugate, which is excreted as such in the urine at the rate of 5–20 ng/day.

Hyperaldosteronism
Physiological
Pregnancy

Peak levels just before delivery. ? increased renin substrate induced by oestrogen? antagonism for aldosterone-binding sites by progesterone.

Pathological
Primary

1. Aldosterone-producing adrenal adenoma. Adrenal vein aldosterone/cortisol ratio increased, with suppression of the contra-lateral gland.
2. Idiopathic adrenal hyperplasia—does not respond to surgery. Following 3 days of 250–300 mmol/day sodium supplements + 0·5 mg fludrocortisone per day, the ECF volume is expanded—aldosterone excretion exceeds 95 per cent upper limit after 3 days (cf. patients with essential hypertension 12·1 nmol/24 h with normal or low plasma renin activity).

Secondary
NON-HYPERTENSIVE

Sodium depletion (osmolality reduced).
Nephrosis ⎫ Hypoproteinaemia results in reduced osmolality
Hepatic cirrhosis ⎭ with consequent aldosterone release.
Congestive cardiac failure—reduced cardiac output results in reduced plasma volume, with consequent aldosterone release.
Idiopathic oedema—reduced plasma volume.
Salt-losing nephritis.
Bartter's syndrome.

HYPERTENSIVE

Malignant hypertension.
Juxtamedullary cell tumour.
Diuretic therapy.

Aldosterone Deficiency

Signs and Symptoms of Aldosterone Deficiency (Severe)

There is urinary wasting of sodium and water, with diminution of the ECF. Plasma potassium levels rise with metabolic acidosis (as hydrogen ions are inadequately excreted). Cardiac output falls progressively until death.

Generalized Adrenocortical Insufficiency

Addison's primary adrenocortical insufficiency.

21-hydroxylase deficiency—glucocorticoids reduced, mineralocorticoids reduced, with increased circulating renin.

Hypopituitarism—resulting in secondary adrenocortical insufficiency.

Selective Aldosterone Deficiency

Primary adrenal gland defect:
18-hydroxylase deficiency.
18-hydroxydehydrogenase deficiency.
(Chronic heparin therapy has been reported as causing atrophy of zona glomerulosa.)

Defect of Aldosterone Control Mechanism

Congenital—primary renal salt retention.
Acquired—chronic renal disease.

BLOOD AMMONIA

Exogenous Sources

The main source of exogenous ammonia is from bacterial and non-bacterial enzymic action on gastrointestinal contents, with release of ammonia in the large bowel, especially the caecum, and to a lesser extent in the stomach.

After ureterosigmoidostomy there is enhanced reabsorption of chloride and ammonium ions derived from chloride and urea excreted in the urine into the large bowel. Some of the ammonium ions are broken down to ammonia and hydrogen ions before absorption.

The portal circulation has a relatively high blood ammonia concentration, derived from the gut contents, and this is detoxicated in the liver, where glutamate and ammonia form glutamine, and aspartate and ammonia form asparagine.

Blood for transfusion contains up to 29·4 µmol/l (50µg/100 ml) at the time of collection, rising to 400 µmol/l (680 µg/100 ml) by the twenty-first day of storage. Fresh blood should therefore be used for patients with liver failure and for infants.

Moderate amounts of ammonia are present in various non-human milk feeds, and these cause increases in the infant's blood ammonia concentration.

Endogenous Sources

Small amounts of ammonia are synthesized in the lungs and liver. Severe hyperammonaemia, particularly after protein feeds (e.g. milk), is almost always due to inborn errors of metabolism in infants (e.g. enzyme deficiency in the Krebs–Henseleit urea cycle).

In adults with severe liver disease, and especially after portacaval anastomosis, blood ammonia levels can rise above 175 µmol/l (300 µg/100 ml) causing severe toxic effects, including convulsions and coma.

The newborn infant can only tolerate much lower levels of blood ammonia, and convulsions may develop when the blood ammonia concentration rises above 60 µmol/l (100 µg/100 ml).

Blood ammonia estimation is difficult and only a limited number of laboratories undertake it. The estimation must be made as soon as the blood sample has been taken. It plays a very important part in the detection of inherited disorders of metabolism in newborn infants.

The ammonia synthesized in the kidney is excreted in the urine as ammonium ion, and does not affect the blood ammonia concentration.

BLOOD AMMONIA
Normal Infant

During the first few weeks of life there is normally a wide variation in blood ammonia concentration varying with the ammonia content of different non-human milk feeds given.
$Mean = 95$ µmol/l (160 µg/100 ml) s.d. $= \pm 41$ µmol/l (69·7 µg/100 ml).

Normal Adult

Normal arterial plasma ammonia $= < 5·88$ µmol/l (< 10 µg/100 ml).
Normal venous plasma ammonia $= < 17·85$ µmol/l (< 30 µg/100 ml).
Normal blood draining gastrointestinal tract = approximately 88 µmol/l (150 µg/100 ml).

Pathological Increase

1 Liver disease
    a Acute hepatic necrosis ⎫ especially after:
    b Terminal cirrhosis   ⎭ i Protein meal.
                                      ii Ammonium chloride load.
                                      iii Portacaval shunt.
                                      iv Resins in the ammonium phase.
2 Congenital enzyme deficiencies, including:
    a Carbamyl phosphate synthetase deficiency.
    b Ornithine transcarbamylase deficiency.
    c Argininosuccinate synthetase deficiency.
    d Arginase deficiency.
    e Congenital lysine intolerance.
3 Haemorrhagic shock.

URINE AMMONIUM

Ammonia is synthesized in the renal tubular cells, with the main sites of production in the distal tubules and the collecting ducts. Once ammonia, which is a very strong base capable of passing freely across membranes, enters the renal tubular lumen, it combines with free hydrogen ions to form lipid-insoluble water-soluble ammonium, trapped as a positively charged ion, and excreted in the urine. When the urine pH is less than 5·0 (10 000 nmol/l of hydrogen ions), both phosphate and ammonia combine with nearly the maximum number of hydrogen ions. Chronic metabolic acidosis enhances transport of glutamine into the renal tubular cell mitochondria specifically.

Of the ammonium excreted in the urine, which is derived from ammonia synthesized in the tubular cells—

1. Forty per cent is derived from the amide group of glutamine, and glutamine is extracted by the tubular cells from the renal blood. The enzyme glutaminase is present in the mitochondria of the tubular cells.

2. Twenty per cent is derived from the amino groups in: (1) Glutamine; (2) Glutamate.

3. Ten per cent is derived from the amino groups in: (1) Alanine; (2) Glycine.

4. Thirty per cent is derived from ammonia which diffuses from the blood into the renal tubular cells. The portal circulation has a relatively high blood ammonia concentration, the ammonia being mostly absorbed from the caecum, where bacterial urease activity splits urea.

Transamination of alpha-ketoglutarate with amino groups from other amino acids generates more glutamate.

The normal hydrogen ion excretion in the adult is 50 per cent in the form of ammonium, and 50 per cent in the form of titratable acid.

Normal Urine Ammonium Excretion

The normal adult output on a normal diet is 30–50 mmol/day. In acidosis up to 500 mmol can be produced and excreted in the urine each day. Gluconeogenesis is promoted in acidosis, removing alpha-ketoglutarate, which may allow increased deamination of glutamine, The rate of renal gluconeogenesis from amino acid residues correlates with the rate of ammonia production in response to acidosis. When a continued ammonium chloride load is given, there is an initial loss of sodium in the urine, followed by potassium exchange and excretion, sparing sodium. This is followed by increased urine ammonium excretion, sparing both sodium and potassium, the result of increased ammonia synthesis. The ammonium in the ammonium chloride load is detoxicated to urea in the liver, releasing chloride and inducing metabolic acidosis. This change takes hours or days to develop, as ammonia synthesis depends on the amount of enzyme present in renal tubular cells, which has to be synthesized, before ammonia can be synthesized. Extraction of glutamine from renal artery blood increases in the kidney within 60 min of an acid load being given.

Increased Urine Ammonium Excretion

1. *Physiological*

   a High meat intake (i.e. increased hydrogen ion release from protein).

   b Starvation (i.e. body protein breakdown). Urine ammonium increases in the first 10 days to 5 × normal, and paradoxical alkaline urine occurs after 6 days.

   c Normal pregnancy during the last 3 months.

2. *Pathological*

   a Acidosis
      i Metabolic.
      ii Respiratory.
   b Hyperaldosteronism.
   c Hypokalaemia.
   d Fanconi syndrome.
   e After ureterosigmoidostomy there is enhanced reabsorption of chloride and ammonium excreted in the urine. The resulting metabolic acidosis increases ammonia synthesis and ammonium excretion.

Decreased Urine Ammonium Excretion

   a Alkalosis
      i Metabolic

   ii Respiratory
  b Rich vegetable diet with low meat content, i.e. alkaline, or only weakly acid urine.
  c Addison's disease.
  d Renal tubular damage affecting the distal tubules, e.g. renal tubular acidosis Type 4, in which the ammonium excretion is inversely proportional to the plasma potassium concentration.
  e Diabetes mellitus treated with phenformin (? of significance in the development of lactic acidosis).
  f Hyperkalaemia. Ammonia synthesis is inhibited by hyperkalaemia.

ANGIOTENSIN II
Source
Angiotensin II is an octapeptide derived from angiotensin I (in turn derived from angiotensinogen), via the actions of renin and converting enzyme. It is found in circulating blood, but a considerable amount is also formed in the kidney, probably in the juxtaglomerular cells. Renin release is the rate-limiting step in angiotensin production.

Actions
1. Angiotensin II stimulates plain muscle and is a very powerful short-acting vasopressor agent. Arteriolar constriction results in raised blood pressure (increasing both diastolic and systolic pressures). The rise in blood pressure is rapid, and lasts for up to 20 min after cessation of an infusion of angiotensin II. Prolonged infusion does not produce a prolonged rise in blood pressure (cf. renin).

Following acute haemorrhage, angiotensin II levels increase, but it has only a minor role in maintenance of blood pressure and probably is more important in the pathway resulting in aldosterone release (which helps to maintain ECF volume). In the coronary circulation, it causes increase in coronary vessel resistance, with reduced coronary artery blood flow.

2. Angiotensin II causes vasoconstriction of the afferent glomerular arterioles in the kidney, greater than of the corresponding efferent arterioles. The glomerular filtration pressure is increased with reduced renal blood flow, resulting in increased renal tubular reabsorption of filtrate (the peritubular capillary pressure being reduced). In consequence the fluid volume excreted is reduced. Angiotensin II probably plays a very important part in the intermittent opening and near-closing of individual nephrons during moderate or reduced fluid volume excretion.

Underperfusion of the kidneys in congestive cardiac failure results in increased renin release, and hence in increased angiotensin I, II and III, with release of aldosterone and subsequent salt and water retention. Renal arterial pressure falls following a fall in ECF volume and/or reduction in effective circulating volume. This is followed by renin release and hence aldosterone release.

3. Angiotensin II stimulates vasoconstrictor neurons centrally, and can cause release of ADH into the circulation. In experimental animals it has been shown that perfusion of angiotensin II into the hypothalamus induces drinking in the conscious animal, and may play a part in the origin of thirst in man.

Elimination

Angiotensin II is rapidly destroyed in the peripheral capillary beds by angiotensinases. It is also converted to angiotensin III, which causes formation and release of aldosterone.

Increased circulating Angiotensin II

1 Essential hypertension.
2 Other forms of hypertension.
3 Renin-secreting juxtaglomerular tumour.
4 Bartter's syndrome—with reduced responsiveness of renal musculature or potassium wasting.
5 Reduced effective circulating volume, e.g. acute haemorrhage.
6 Sympathetic nerve system stimulation.
7 Hyponatraemia.
8 Potassium restriction in diet (with increased renin release and reduced basal renal blood flow).

Reduced circulating Angiotensin II

1 Primary hyperaldosteronism (Conn's syndrome).
2 Anephric patient.

ANION GAP

Total plasma cations = total plasma anions.
Anion gap (Sodium mmol/l) − (Chloride mmol/l + Bicarbonate mmol/l) = 12 mmol/l (range in normal subject = 8–16 mmol/l)

Total plasma cations = sodium + potassium + unmeasured cations.
Since potassium levels in plasma do not change greatly, potassium is usually missed from the calculation.

Unmeasured cations:
Potassium (see above).
Magnesium ⎱ not usually included in basic 'electrolyte'
Calcium ⎰ request, and not changing over a wide range.
Lithium (therapeutic levels rarely exceed 1·5 mmol/l).
Total plasma anions = chloride + bicarbonate + unmeasured anions.
Unmeasured anions:
Phosphate.
Sulphate.
Creatinine.
Protein (protein can exist either as anion or cation—zwitterion).
Organic acids (normally in low concentrations):
Lactic acid.
Beta-hydroxybutyrate/acetoacetate.

High Anion Gap
1. *Increased Unmeasured Anions*

a Ketoacidosis
  Starvation
  Alcoholic
  Diabetes mellitus
b Uraemia—increased phosphate and sulphate retention, plus other undefined anions.
c Lactic acidosis—including
  ethylene glycol poisoning
  paraldehyde
  fructose administration
  sorbitol
  xylitol
  phenformin
  glycogen storage disease Type I
  fructose-1, 6-diphosphatase deficiency
  methylmalonic aciduria
d Exogenous anions
  salicylate
  antibiotics (e.g. penicillin, carbenicillin)
  formate in methanol poisoning
e Rhabdomyolysis—unidentified plasma anions.

2. *Decreased Measured Anions*

a Severe dehydration.
b Diuretic therapy.
c Combined diuretic and steroid therapy.

3. Decreased Unmeasured Cations

Decreases in potassium, calcium and magnesium to the lower limits compatible with life can cause an increased anion gap. In gross magnesium deficiency, all these three cations are decreased.

4. Laboratory Error

Plasma sodium incorrectly reported as *raised, or incorrectly low chloride* and/or bicarbonate, can give a spurious increased anion gap.

If the anion gap exceeds $0.5 \times$ bicarbonate concentration $+ 16$ mmol/l (i.e. 16 mmol/l is the normal upper limit of the anion gap) a presumptive diagnosis of organic acidosis is justified.

Low Anion Gap

1. Increased Cations

a Severe hypernatremia—volume contraction frequent, with poor tissue perfusion, azotaemia and lactic acidosis.

b Increased unmeasured cations

Potassium.
Magnesium [R].
Calcium.
Lithium.
Gammaglobulins (proteins can act as anions) paraproteins.

2. Decreased Unmeasured Anions

Bromism [R].
Low plasma albumin.

3. Laboratory Error

Incorrectly reported hyponatraemia.

Incorrectly reported increased plasma chloride and/or bicarbonate.

(Unfortunately laboratory error is the commonest cause of low anion gap.)

4. When a blood sample is collected near to an intravenous infusion of isotonic or hypertonic sodium chloride solution, a factitious low anion gap results.

Normal Anion Gap

Normal Anion Gap with Normal or Raised Plasma Potassium

1   Hyperalimentation.

2 Post-hypercapnoea.
3 Rapid hydration (dilutional acidosis). In a volume expansion state there is reduced proximal renal tubule reabsorption of sodium and bicarbonate (a similar occurrence in mineralocorticoid deficiency) resulting in a normal anion gap acidosis.
4 Hypoaldosteronism
   Hyporeninism.
   Selective or general adrenal deficiency.
5 Oral ammonium chloride or calcium chloride.
6 Lysine or arginine hydrochloride therapy.
7 Early uraemic acidosis.

Normal Anion Gap with Reduced Plasma Potassium

1 Gastrointestinal
   Diarrhoea.
   Pancreatic fistula.
2 Ureteral surgery
   Ureterosigmoidostomy.
   Obstructed ileal bladder.
3 Renal tubular acidosis
   Proximal (Type 2).
   Distal (Type 1).

ANTIDIURETIC HORMONE (ADH)

Production and Storage

ADH is an octapeptide with a biological half-life of 16–20 min, synthesized in the supraoptic and paraventricular nuclei of the hypothalamus. It is carried via the supraopticohypophyseal tract and stored in the posterior pituitary gland with its carrier proteins, neurophysins. It is thought possible that the neurophysins affect the renal tubular transport of the hormone.

Action of ADH on the Posterior Nephron

The collecting duct in the absence of ADH is impermeable to water. Solute is reabsorbed, and a dilute urine containing 40–50 mosmol/kg is produced and excreted. When ADH is released, it binds to receptors on the collecting tubules, adenylate cyclase is activated, producing ATP and hence cyclic-AMP. Also a phosphorylation reaction occurs, and as a result, water flow is stimulated across the luminal membrane. Water leaves the tubular lumen and re-enters the circulation. ADH requires 30–60 min to exert an effect on sodium transport.

Factors affecting ADH Release

When plasma osmolality increases by 1–2 per cent, ADH is secreted, whereas when plasma osmolality falls by 1–2 per cent ADH release is suppressed. During a fluid fast, a loss of 1 per cent in body weight is accompanied by a 3 per cent rise in plasma osmolality. Circulatory volume change receptors in the carotid sinus, aortic arch, left atrium and the large veins, if they detect a decrease greater than − 10 per cent, trigger release of ADH, and if they detect an increase greater than + 10 per cent they suppress ADH release. When the apparent decrease in volume is greater than − 10 per cent ADH is released regardless of the associated osmolality.

Plasma osmolality > 292 mosmol/kg or plasma sodium > 144 mmol/l are the lowest levels at which in normal adults there is an invariable rise in plasma vasopressin and an increase in urine concentration.

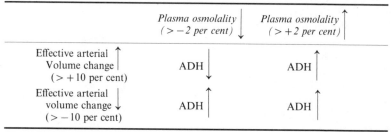

ADH release responses to (a) plasma osmolality, and (b) effective arterial volume changes.

Non-specific Stimuli for ADH Release

General anaesthesia ⎫ i.e. it is not sensible to expect a diuresis after
Trauma ⎬ a surgical operation, even if fluid has been
Surgery (= trauma) ⎭ given intravenously.
Inflammatory disease of the CNS
Vincristine
Clofibrate
Nicotine
Chlorpropamide
Alpha-adrenergic impulses

Drugs which Impair Renal Water Excretion, by stimulating ADH Release

Barbiturates
Carbamazepine
Chlorpropamide

Clofibrate (also potentiates submaximal levels of ADH)
Isoproterenol
Morphine
Nicotine
Vincristine

Other Drugs which Impair Renal Water Excretion

Acetoaminophen
Cyclophosphamide, associated with abnormal water excretion
Indomethacin—inhibits prostaglandins
Tolbutamide
Most of these drugs have caused hyponatraemia. Many have been used to treat partial diabetes insipidus.

Inappropriate Absence of ADH Activity

Diabetes insipidus
Brain injury affecting the area around the posterior pituitary
Nephrogenic diabetes insipidus
   Primary
   Secondary, with:
      Hypokalaemia
      Hypercalcaemia
      Osmotic diuresis
      Sickle-cell disease
      Amyloidosis.
Chronic nephritis.
Recovery phase following acute tubular necrosis.
Recovery phase following relief of urinary tract obstruction.

Pharmacological Inhibition of ADH Activity on Collecting Tubules

Demeclocycline therapy—impairment of cAMP production.
Lithium carbonate—interferes with the peripheral action of ADH on renal tubules.
After penthrane anaesthesia (rare).

'Distal Trickle' Effect

When the GFR is low, there is increased proximal tubular absorption of the smaller glomerular filtrate. Reduced luminal fluid reaches the ascending loop of Henle. The luminal fluid passes slowly through the distal tubules in partial equilibrium with the renal interstitium. A moderately concentrated urine is produced in the absence of ADH activity.

Reduced Responsiveness to ADH

Obstructive uropathy.

Amyloid disease.

Sjögren's syndrome, with immunological tubulo-interstitial disease. Polyuria precedes failure.

Hypokalaemia with potassium depletion.

Hypercalcaemia—reduced capacity to form cAMP following the action of ADH on the distal tubular cells.

Sickle-cell disease—sickling of red cells in medulla causes reduction in blood supply and hence progressive damage;—decreased ability to maintain high concentrations of sodium chloride in the medullary interstitium.

Postrenal transplant.

Medullary cystic disease.

Pyelonephritis.

Radiation nephritis.

Light-chain nephropathy—polyuria.

Multiple myeloma (light chains affecting tubules, causing polyuria).

Sarcoidosis—may be associated with hypercalcaemia.

Congenital nephrogenic diabetes insipidus.

BASE EXCESS/DEFICIT

Base Excess = the amount of acid required to titrate blood pH back to pH 7·4 at a P_{CO_2} of 5·4 kPa (40 mmHg) at 37 °C.

Base Excess = the difference between the observed total buffer base and the 'normal' buffer base allowing for the haemoglobin concentration.

Negative Base Excess (Base Deficit) = the amount of alkali required to titrate the blood pH back to pH 7·4 at P_{CO_2} of 5·4 kPa (40 mmHg) at 37 °C.

Treatment

Treat the cause.

A calculation has been given in which the amount of base (acid) requried for correction = 0·3 × deficit (excess) in mmol/l × body weight in kg. Unfortunately this estimation is unreliable and encourages overenthusiastic treatment. It is much better to give 100–200 mmol of bicarbonate for deficit, or acid for excess, intravenously over a period of at least 5 min. The blood pH, bicarbonate, P_{CO_2}, sodium and potassium concentrations should be checked after 30 min, and further treatment should be given empirically as necessary and based on these results.

In acidosis it is important to increase a low plasma pH to above pH 7·2, when the respiratory drive is greatly reduced towards normal.

BICARBONATE

Carbon dioxide produced by tissue metabolism enters the blood and is dissolved in the plasma in proportion to the Pa_{CO_2}. Carbonic acid is formed by a reversible reaction, with very rapid development of equilibrium because of the general body distribution of the enzyme carbonic anhydrase:

$$CO_2 + H_2O \rightleftharpoons H_2CO_3$$

The fixed ratio of dissolved carbon dioxide to carbonic acid is 800 : 1 and the total (dissolved carbon dioxide + carbonic acid) is regarded for practical purposes as carbonic acid. Plasma carbonic acid is therefore directly proportional to Pa_{CO_2}. When 5 ml of carbon dioxide are added from the tissues to 100 ml blood, 0·5 ml is in solution and 3·5 ml are carried as bicarbonate, the plasma pH falling from 7·40 to 7·36. Of the 50 ml of carbon dioxide in each 100 ml of arterial blood, 3 ml are dissolved, 3 ml are combined with carbamino compounds, and 44 ml circulate as bicarbonate ion.

$$H_2CO_3 \rightleftharpoons HCO_3 + H^+$$

Hence

$$[H^+] = \frac{K[H_2CO_3]}{[HCO_3^-]} \quad \text{where K is the Dissociation Constant.}$$

Since the amount of carbonic acid and dissolved carbon dioxide is proportional to the P_{CO_2}

$$[H^+] = \frac{K[a \cdot Pa_{CO_2}]}{[HCO_3^-]}$$

where a is the solubility coefficient for carbon dioxide in plasma and $K = 24 \times 10^{-9}$.

$$H^+ \text{ (nmol/l)} = \left(\frac{24 \times Pa_{CO_2} \text{ (kPa)} \times 7·5}{HCO_3^- \text{ (mmol/l)}} \right) = \left(\frac{24 \times Pa_{CO_2} \text{ (mmHg)}}{HCO_3^- \text{ (mmol/l)}} \right)$$

or

$$pH = 6·1 + \log_{10}\left(\frac{HCO_3^- \text{ (mmol/l)}}{0·0301 \times Pa_{CO_2} \text{ (mmHg)}} \right)$$

$$= 6·1 + \log_{10}\left(\frac{HCO_3^- \text{ (mmol/l)}}{0·0301 \times 7·5 \times Pa_{CO_2}(kPa)} \right)$$

The plasma pH (or plasma hydrogen ion concentration) reflects the Pa_{CO_2}, and the bicarbonate concentration in the ECF varying with the ratio of Pa_{CO_2}/HCO_3^-. While carbon dioxide diffuses freely and rapidly across cell membranes, bicarbonate and hydrogen ions only diffuse and equilibrate slowly, for example across the blood–brain barrier.

Body Distribution

Plasma—26 mmol/l (24–32).

ISF—approximately 31 mmol/l.

ICF—approximately 8 mmol/l.

CSF—1–2 mmol/l less than the equivalent plasma concentration. Equilibration after a change in plasma concentration takes hours (cf. $Pa_{CO_2}/CSF P_{CO_2}$).

Saliva—20–60 mmol/l (50 mmol/24 h).

Bile—20–40 mmol/l (40 mmol/24 h).

Pancreatic juice—80–120 mmol/l (120 mmol/24 h).

Intestinal juice—variable.

Renal Treatment of Bicarbonate

No bicarbonate is lost in the urine in health, unless a bicarbonate load is given. When the plasma bicarbonate level exceeds 25–27 mmol/l, bicarbonate begins to appear in the urine.

Each day bicarbonate freely filtered by the glomeruli from the plasma enters the proximal convoluted tubule at the rate of 4500 mmol HCO_3^-, and 90 per cent of this load is reabsorbed in the proximal tubule. Hydrogen ions are secreted into the lumen in exchange for reabsorbed sodium ions, and they combine with bicarbonate ions to form carbonic acid. The carbonic acid dissociates into carbon dioxide and water. Carbon dioxide rapidly diffuses back into the plasma. The rate at which the kidney returns bicarbonate to the body fluid in this way is equivalent to the rate at which sodium ions are exchanged for hydrogen ions.

1. *Proximal Renal Tubule Bicarbonate Reabsorption*

Increased

Increased bicarbonate load in GFR with increased arterial Pa_{CO_2}, and hypokalaemia.

Diminished effective arterial volume.

Volume depletion associated with chloride depletion.

Decreased PTH activity.

Hypocalcaemia.
Hypophosphataemia.

Decreased

Reduced $Paco_2$.
Hyperkalaemia.
Increased EAV.
Increased PTH activity—resulting in increased excretion of sodium,
potassium, bicarbonate and water.
Hypercalcaemia.
Hyperphosphataemia.
Renal tubular acidosis, Type 2.

2. Loop of Henle
Minimal bicarbonate exchange.

3. Distal Renal Tubule and Collecting Duct
Remainder of bicarbonate normally reabsorbed during the generation
or maintenance of the steep luminal–peritubular hydrogen ion gradient
by hydrogen ion secretion into the luminal fluid. This bicarbonate
reabsorption is impaired in renal tubular acidosis, Type I.

Plasma Bicarbonate
1. Reduced Bicarbonate
Primary Fall

Metabolic acidosis—if $Paco_2$ higher than expected, then this suggests
associated respiratory acidosis;—if $Paco_2$ lower than expected, then
this suggests associated respiratory alkalosis.

Secondary (Compensatory) Fall
Respiratory alkalosis.

2. Increased Plasma Bicarbonate
Primary Increase—metabolic alkalosis
Secondary Increase (Compensatory)—respiratory alkalosis.

Signs and Symptoms of bicarbonate deficit
Deep rapid breathing
Shortness of breath on exertion

Weakness
Stupor
Coma
Urine pH $<6\cdot0$
Plasma pH $<7\cdot35$

Bicarbonate Replacement Therapy

When bicarbonate is given, 50 per cent is 'dissipated' by hydrogen ions relinquished by other buffers, i.e. calculations for replacement therapy are not reliable.

Since transfer of hydrogen ions from the ECF to ICF takes more than 2 h, complete equilibration after bicarbonate infusion takes at least 2 h. Rapid correction of metabolic acidosis with bicarbonate is dangerous. Hyperventilation due to raised hydrogen ion concentration (low pH) decreases and the plasma Paco$_2$ rises. Carbon dioxide rapidly diffuses into the CSF, where CSF hydrogen ion concentration rises (further fall in pH) as carbonic acid and hence bicarbonate and free hydrogen ions are formed. This results in convulsions and coma.

Bicarbonate induces cellular uptake of potassium, and is used in the treatment of hyperkalaemia, but the mechanism of this is not yet understood.

Plasma Bicarbonate and pK

When a weak acid HA in aqueous solution partially dissociates, $HA \rightleftharpoons H^+ + A^-$ the Dissociation Constant K is defined as $[H^+][A^-]/[HA]$ and pK is defined (by analogy with pH) as $-\log_{10} K$. Plasma bicarbonate can be measured directly by tonometry. Alternatively, many instruments measure Paco$_2$ and plasma pH, calculating either the 'actual' plasma bicarbonate, or the 'standard' bicarbonate (with plasma adjusted to a Pco$_2$ of $5\cdot4$ kPa (40 mmHg) at NTP and 37 °C), using the Henderson-Hasselbalch equation and assuming the pK for bicarbonate to be $6\cdot1$.

Discrepancies have been found between these three different results for plasma bicarbonate, and it has been found that the pK can vary from $5\cdot87$ to $6\cdot43$ in acute severe illness. Variations in calculated plasma bicarbonate levels occur as a result.

1. Variation in plasma ionic strength, the pK increasing with reduction in plasma ionic strength.

2. Variations in the amount of carbon dioxide held on carbamino compounds, with wide variation in plasma pH, and protein and non-protein nitrogen concentration.

3. Variation in the solubility coefficient for carbon dioxide in plasma. The pK varies inversely with body temperature.

a. Overestimation of Plasma Bicarbonate (Calculated)

Low pK results in increased $\log_{10}$ (Bicarbonate/$P\text{CO}_2$)
  i Alkalosis.
  ii Hyperpyrexia.
  iii Hypernatraemia.
e.g. overestimation would occur in metabolic alkalosis with hypernatraemia and hyperpyrexia.

b. Underestimation of Plasma Bicarbonate (Calculated)

High pK results in reduced $\log_{10}$ (Bicarbonate/$P\text{CO}_2$)
  i Acidosis.
  ii Hypothermia.
  iii Hyponatraemia.
e.g. underestimation in severe diabetic ketoacidosis with hyponatraemia and hypothermia. These possible discrepancies are probably clinically unimportant, since correction of plasma bicarbonate excess or deficit is by direct observation of response to therapy, rather than adherence to a 'correction' formula.

BLOOD–BRAIN BARRIER

The neurons of the brain are separated from the blood by:
1. The capillary endothelial cell layer. In the brain capillaries the endothelial cells have no gaps between them. Each endothelial cell is attached to all contiguous cells by two bands of 'tight junctions'.
2. Acellular basement membrane.
3. An almost complete layer of end-foot processes arising from astrocytes. Therefore all molecules have to pass through the luminal and antiluminal cell membranes, and cannot pass between the cells. Lipophilic molecules, such as oxygen and carbon dioxide, pass across the boundary easily.

Hydrophilic molecules, such as glucose, ketones, amino acids require special transport mechanisms. In hypoglycaemia, glucose only passes across slowly.
4. There is a further metabolic barrier in the form of an almost complete glial cell layer, and the astrocytes rapidly metabolize ammonia and medium-chain length free fatty acids, which are neurotoxic.

BUFFERS
Buffer Systems

An acid can dissociate to produce hydrogen ions (H^+ protons), and a strong acid is highly dissociated in aqueous solutions, whereas a weak acid is only slightly dissociated.

A weak acid in the presence of its salt forms a buffer system which resists change in hydrogen ion concentration when hydrogen ions are added, the change in hydrogen ion concentration being less than if all the added hydrogen ions remained free. The missing hydrogen ions are removed, the stronger acid being replaced by weaker acid, with reduction in free hydrogen ions:

$$HCl \longrightarrow H^+ + Cl^- \quad \text{(i.e. a strong acid almost completely dissociated).}$$

$$H^+ + Cl^- + NaHCO_3 \rightleftharpoons H_2CO_3 + NaCl.$$

Strong acid + (Strong base-weak acid) $\longrightarrow$ salt (Strong acid-base) + weaker acid.

$$pH = pK + \log \frac{\text{Dissociated acid}}{\text{Undissociated acid}}$$

where pK = negative logarithm of the dissociation constant of the acid. The buffer's greatest capacity for 'mopping up' free hydrogen ions is when:

$$[A^-] = [HA] \quad \text{and} \quad pH = pKa$$
$$H^+ + \text{buffer} \rightleftharpoons H \text{ Buffer and 50 per cent of the buffer}$$
is in the H buffer form.

The normal body buffering systems cope with the excess of free hydrogen ions produced during normal body metabolism, maintaining the normal plasma pH between 7·45 and 7·35 (35 and 45 nmol/l).

Weak acids	Stronger bases	System
H_2CO_3	HCO_3^-	Bicarbonate
		35% of capacity (+ 18% in red cells)
HHb	B^+Hb	Haemoglobin
		35% of total capacity
$B^+H_2PO_4$	$B_2^+HPO_4^{2-}$	Inorganic phosphate
B^+RHPO_4	$B_2^+RPO_4$	Organic phosphate
HPr	B^+Pr^-	Protein

Bone buffer—calcium phosphate enters ECF when the ECF pH falls. Phosphate, creatinine and urate act as weak buffers, and accept free hydrogen ions for excretion in the urine.

pK for bicarbonate system = 6·1.

pK for phosphate system = 6·8.

pK for protein system = 6·8.

pK for haemoglobin system = 6·8.

Bicarbonate System

$$pH = 6\cdot1 + \log\frac{[HCO_3^-]}{[H_2CO_3]} = 6\cdot1 = \log\frac{[HCO_3]}{[Pco_2 \times 0\cdot225\,Kp]}$$

$$= 6\cdot1 + \log\frac{[HCO_3]}{[Pco_2 \times 0\cdot03\,mmHg]}$$

$H_2CO_3 \rightleftharpoons$ total CO_2 in plasma $\rightleftharpoons HCO_3^-$ + dissolved CO_2 + carbonic acid.

(Dissolved CO_2 + carbonic acid) $\propto$ prevailing Pco_2.

Pco_2 of 40 mmHg = dissolved $CO_2 + H_2CO_3$ of 1·2 mmol/l $(40 \times 0\cdot03 = 1\cdot2)$.

Total CO_2 of 25 mmol/l at Pco_2 of 40 mmHG = $HCO_3^- = 25 - 1\cdot2 = 23\cdot8$.

Urine Buffer System

Titratable acid = 10–30 mmol/day (mainly phosphate).
= amount of alkali needed to titrate urine back to pH of plasma.

Urine buffer—pK must be greater than the minimum attainable urine pH.

—pK must be less than the plasma pH.

Phosphate System

At pH 7·4 $HPO_4^{2-} : H_2PO_4^- = 4:1$; at pH 4·4 this ratio become 1:400.

Urate System

At pH 7·4 urate : uric acid = 40:1; at pH 4·4 this ratio becomes 1:40.

Creatinine System

At pH 7·4 creatinine : creatine = 250:1; at pH 4·4 this ratio becomes 1:4.

On a normal diet the urine pH averages about 6·0, when phosphate accepts free hydrogen ions, but urate and creatinine are not very effective.

In severe diabetic or starvation ketoacidosis, aceto-acetic acid and beta-hydroxybutyric acid systems can buffer free hydrogen ions, as their pKs are 3·6 and 4·4 respectively.

Less important in human physiology and pathology, base can accept hydrogen ion, and alkalis dissociate to produce free hydroxyl ions

(OH$^-$). Similar buffering systems can occur to reduce the effect of added hydroxyl ions to a buffer system, e.g.

$$\text{strong base} + \text{weak acid} \rightleftharpoons \text{salt} + \text{water.}$$
$$\text{NaOH} + \text{H}_2\text{CO}_3 \rightleftharpoons \text{Na}_2\text{HCO}_3 + \text{H}_2\text{O}.$$

CALCITONIN, THYROCALCITONIN

Calcitonin, 32 amino-acid residue polypeptide, mol. wt 3500 daltons, is secreted by parafollicular thyroid cells (C cells) sparsely concentrated in the midportion of the lateral lobes of the thyroid gland. The normal plasma concentration is 3–30 pmol/l, but the hormone is not detectable in the blood of 30 per cent of normal adults.

Action

A dose of calcitonin causes a transient increase in the number of osteoblasts and in the rate of bone formation at sites of recent bone resorption. After long-term treatment with calcitonin bone formation is depressed.

Renal excretion of calcium, magnesium, phosphate, sodium and potassium is increased. It also possibly affects absorption of calcium and phosphate from the intestinal tract. The hormone binds to specific receptors, distinct from PTH receptors, followed by adenylate cyclase activation, and then cAMP generation.

Increased Calcitonin

Patients with thyrocalcitonin-secreting medullary carcinoma of the thyroid develop hypocalcaemia without other electrolyte disturbances. (The renal action of the hormone cannot be important.)

In dialysis patients, those with normal plasma alkaline phosphatase activity have lower immunoreactive parathyroid hormone (iPTH) levels and higher immunoreactive calcitonin (iCT) levels than those patients with raised plasma alkaline phosphatase activity.

Therapeutics

Calcitonin is used in the treatment of hypercalcaemia arising from excessive release of calcium from bone. There is a significant fall in plasma calcium within 4–12 h of injection, but never severe hypocalcaemia. Escape from the hypocalcaemic effects of calcitonin occurs after days to weeks of continuous calcitonin dosage. In the prolonged treatment of Paget's osteitis deformans with calcitonin, bone turn-over is reduced, as is the number of osteoclasts. There is no severe hypocalcaemia or marked increase in plasma PTH. There is suppression of recruitment of new osteoclasts from precursor cells.

CALCIUM

Dietary Content
Milk, diary products and meat. Average intake 20–30 mmol/day.

Absorption
Absorption of calcium is maximal in the duodenum. $1,25\text{-}(OH)_2D_3$ stimulates the absorption of calcium, magnesium and phosphate from the intestine, facilitated by lactose and protein. Absorption is inhibited by phosphates, oxalates and phytates. The proportion absorbed from the gastrointestinal tract is directly related to the body's requirement for calcium.

Function
1 Bone structure—bone modelling, resorption and deposition involve 5 mmol/day, with most resorption occurring at rest overnight.
2 Neuromuscular transmission—the influence on muscle potential includes its influence of the cardiac potential.
3 Secretion of endocrine and exocrine glands, i.e. it is a 'messenger', bound in cells to calcium-binding protein until stimulation.
4 Enzyme reactions, e.g. essential for alkaline phosphatase activity.
5 Complement activation.
6 Fibrinolysis activation.
7 Plasma clotting factor activation.
8 Release of bound intracellular calcium in platelets is essential for the 'release' reaction of platelets during the development of a platelet thrombus. Ionized calcium is essential for platelet adhesion to collagen and for platelet aggregation.

Body Distribution
Of the total body calcium 99 per cent is 'insoluble', but the surface crystals in bone are exchangeable with the ECF calcium.

1. *Plasma Calcium*
Normal mean value = 2·4 mmol/l (9·6 mg/dl), range 2·2–2·6 mmol/l (8·8–10·4 mg/dl). The plasma calcium concentration rises slightly after meals, and is slightly higher when the subject is in the upright position,

when compared with results obtained when the subject is recumbent. Plasma calcium varies directly with the plasma albumin, and is increased when blood is taken using a tourniquet restricting blood flow (and increasing plasma albumin).

2. ECF Calcium

Concentration approximately 2·5 mmol/l (10 mg/100 ml).
—47 per cent ionized.
—13·5 per cent non-ionized but ultrafiltrable, and able to diffuse across the capillary wall (complexed with carbonate and phosphate).
—39·5 per cent protein-bound.

An increase in pH by 0·1 unit results in an increase in protein-bound calcium of 0·043 mmol/l (0·17 mg/100 ml) at the expense of ionized calcium.

A decrease of pH by 0·1 unit results in a fall in protein-bound calcium of 0·043 mmol/l (0·17 mg/100 ml) with a corresponding increase in ionized calcium.

3. CSF Calcium

CSF calcium = 1·15 mmol/l.

4. Sweat Calcium

Normal sweat involves the loss of up to 0·375 mmol/day, but during exertion in extreme heat more than 2·5 mmol/l can be lost in the sweat.

5. Lactation and Pregnancy

In pregnancy and during lactation the bodily requirement is 100–125 mmol/day (0·4–0·5 g/day).

6. ICF Calcium

Intracellular calcium concentration = 1 mmol/l (2 mEq/l, 4 mg/100 ml), mostly complexed and chemically inert (see Functions).

Renal Excretion

Forty per cent of the plasma calcium is bound to plasma albumin and not filtered. More than 98 per cent of the glomerular filtered calcium is reabsorbed by the renal tubules. Fifty to fifty-five per cent is reabsorbed in the proximal tubules in proportion to sodium reabsorption. Twenty to thirty per cent is reabsorbed in the loop of Henle, again in proportion to the sodium load reabsorbed. A further 12–23 per cent is reabsorbed in the distal renal tubules by mechanisms unrelated to sodium reabsorption. A total of 2·5–8·75 mmol are excreted in the urine each day normally on an average diet.

Increased Urine Calcium Excretion

1 Increased EAV.
2 Raised plasma calcium concentration.
3 Hormone action.
   a Calcitonin.
   b Human growth hormone.
   c Thyroxine.
   d Glucocorticoids.
4 Acidosis
   a Metabolic acidosis.
   b Respiratory acidosis.
5 Phosphate depletion.
6 Diuretic action
   a Frusemide.
   b Ethacrynic acid.
   c Mercurial diuretics.
   d Osmotic diuretics.

Decreased Urine Calcium Excretion

1 Decreased EAV.
2 Hypocalcaemia.
3 Hormone action—parathyroid hormone.
4 Vitamin D.
5 Alkalosis
   a Metabolic alkalosis.
   b Respiratory alkalosis.
6 Phosphate excess.
7 Diuretic action: thiazide diuretics. Thiazide diuretics have been used with dietary sodium supplements to prevent hypercalcaemia in 'stone formers'.

Faecal Calcium Excretion

1 Unabsorbed dietary calcium.
2 Shed gastrointestinal epithelial cells.
3 Digestive juices. A total of approximately 8 litre/day are secreted and reabsorbed, with recycling of 10 mmol (400 mg) calcium each day.

Hypercalcaemia

Signs and Symptoms

1 Anorexia, nausea and lethargy.
2 Weight loss.
3 Polydipsia and polyuria, including nocturia.
4 Muscle hypotonicity.
5 Azotaemia.
6 Bone cavitation with deep bone pain, if there is rapid bone resorption.
7 Flank pain and signs and symptoms of renal tract stone, a stone has developed as a result of increased urinary calcium concentration.
8 In hypercalcaemia, calcium is precipitated between and across nephrons, and as a fine 'dusting' of tubule cells and their basement membrane. Early lesions are in the collecting ducts, distal tubules and ascending loops of Henle.

There is a profound impairment of the kidney's ability to concentrate urine (this may also occur in the presence of hypercalciuria with normal plasma calcium concentration).

In hypercalcaemia (except when due to primary hyperparathyroidism) there is increased hydrogen ion excretion, with increased urine ammonium, and a low urine pH, with increased plasma bicarbonate and a tendency for plasma pH to rise. Gastric hydrogen ion secretion is also increased. On the other hand, parathyroid hormone inhibits hydrogen ion excretion, and plasma bicarbonate falls with an equivalent rise in plasma chloride.

Causes

1 Hyperparathyroidism (serum calcium increased with low plasma inorganic phosphate)
    a Idiopathic
    b Familial [AD]
        i Werner's (Type I)—associated with pituitary tumours and tumours of pancreatic islet cells.
        ii Sipple's (Type II)—associated with medullary carcinoma of the thyroid and phaeochromocytoma.
2 Malignancy (serum calcium and inorganic phosphate increased)
    a Direct destruction of bone, with calcium release.
    b Tumour releases PTH or PTH-like substance.
    c Release of osteoclast-stimulating activity factor.
    d Production of prostaglandin E causing bone resorption.
    e Vitamin D-like sterols released by the tumour.
3 Some patients on thiazide diuretics.

Treatment

1. Correct any hypernatremia by giving 5 per cent glucose intravenously, followed by 0·45 per cent sodium chloride + 20–30 mmol potassium chloride per litre, at the rate of 6–12 litres per 24 h, with frusemide every 4–6 h to ensure diuresis, if there is a reasonable urine flow.
2. Glucocorticoids. If the hypercalcaemia is due to primary hyperparathyroidism, glucocorticoids are ineffective.
3. Increase phosphate intake.
4. Calcitonin.
5. Mithramycin.
6. Dialysis in desperation.
7. Sequestrene (EDTA) is transient in action and is also toxic, and therefore not useful.

Alternatively, 1 litre of 0·9 per cent sodium chloride solution given every 6 h for 48 h ensures that the patient is hydrated without a forced sodium diuresis. Two litres of 0·9 per cent saline daily are then given until a stable, steady and safe plasma calcium value is reached. Calcitonin and mithramycin are held in reserve in case of clinical deterioration. The saline infusion removes the drive to increased sodium reabsorption in dehydration, with obligate calcium reabsorption. Potassium supplements are not often necessary.

Hypocalcaemia
Signs and Symptoms
1 *Neuromuscular*

Muscle cramps, including abdominal cramps.
Tetany, carpopedal spasm (Chvostek's and Trousseau's signs).
Tingling of the circumoral area.
Tingling and numbness of fingers.
Laryngeal stridor.
Hyperactive reflexes.
Extrapyramidal signs.
Epileptiform seizures.

2 *Mental Changes*

Increased emotional lability.
Depression.
Psychosis.

3 *ECG Changes*

Prolonged Q-T secondary to prolongation of the S-T segment.

4 *Basal Ganglia Calcification*
Hypoparathyroidism.
Pseudohypoparathyroidism.

5 *Skin*
The skin becomes thin and dry. Moniliasis is common. There is loss of hair.

6 *Eyes*
Cataracts.
Keratitis.
Conjunctivitis.

Causes
1. Plasma albumin reduced. Total plasma albumin reduced, and protein-bound calcium falls, but ionized calcium concentration remains normal unless the plasma pH rises above normal, e.g. (*a*) Nephrosis; (*b*) Cirrhosis; (*c*) Malnutrition.
2. Hypoparathyroidism (serum calcium low with raised inorganic phosphate). Reduced circulating parathyroid hormone with reduced resorption of calcium from bone, increased phosphate retention due to reduced renal phosphate excretion. There is also decreased production of 1,25-$(OH)_2D_3$ leading to reduced intestinal absorption of calcium.
    a Idiopathic
       i Idiopathic
          Sporadic
          Familial—infantile [XR]; adolescent [AR].
       ii Associated with thymic aplasia and immune deficiency state—Di George's syndrome.
    b Surgical removal of parathyroid glands
       i Deliberate planned surgery.
       ii Accidental removal of parathyroid glands during thyroidectomy.
3. Associated with
    a Adrenal hyperplasia.
    b Hypogonadism.
    c Thyroiditis (Hashimoto's disease).
    d Pernicious anaemia—depression protein synthesis.
    e Diabetes mellitus.
    f Malabsorption syndrome.
    g Renal failure (low calcium with increased inorganic phosphate)

4. Pseudohypoparathyroidism:
   a Bone and kidney resists PTH action (Type I).
   b Normal response to PTH by cyclic-AMP release, but with no increase in phosphate excretion. ? cyclic-AMP receptor defect.
   c Defective form of PTH hormone released.
   d Renal resistance to the action of PTH, but with normal bone response to PTH action. Increased plasma inorganic phosphate concentration is followed by hypocalcaemia, with defective production of $1,25\text{-}(OH)_2D_3$.
5. Vitamin D deficiency (serum calcium and inorganic phosphate low). There is poor intestinal absorption of calcium from the diet, with decreased resorption of calcium from bone. This results in secondary hyperparathyroidism with low plasma inorganic phosphate levels and a low (calcium × phosphate) product, causing osteomalacia and rickets.
6. Miscellaneous
   a Hypomagnesaemia.
   b Neonatal hypocalcaemia
       Vitamin D deficiency.
       Excessively high phosphate intake in cow's milk.
       Mother receiving treatment with PTH immediately before birth.
   c Miscellaneous
       Massive rapid blood transfusion (excess citrate).
       Calcitonin release after thyroid surgery.
       Osteoblastic metastases [R].
       Burns—the total plasma calcium and ionized calcium concentrations fall after severe burns, and there is increased excretion of calcium in the urine. It is thought that there is an abnormality in PTH release, since there is no rise in circulating PTH, even though the ionized calcium levels are low.

Treatment

1. Urgent treatment:
Calcium gluconate (10 ml of 10 per cent solution) = 2·25 mmol calcium.
Calcium chloride (10 ml of 10 per cent solution) = 9 mmol calcium.
Up to a maximum of 50 mmol of calcium can be given at a rate not faster than 1·25 mmol/min. The plasma calcium concentration should then be checked.
2. Slower oral treatment:
Calcium gluconate tablets containing 2·25 mmol calcium per tablet.

CARBON DIOXIDE

The normal adult generates 14–20 moles of carbon dioxide each day, which is carried to the lungs and expired. During severe exercise the production rate of carbon dioxide increases ten-fold. Carbon dioxide is produced in the ICF in the tissues, and there is a constant flow of carbon dioxide from the cells into the ISF and hence into the plasma, to reach the pulmonary capillaries. Carbon dioxide diffuses rapidly across cell membranes. Of the carbon dioxide 799/800ths is carried dissolved in the plasma water, while 1/800th is converted to carbonic acid.

$$\frac{CO_2}{H_2CO_3} = \frac{800}{1}.$$

Inside the erythrocytes the enzyme carbonic anhydrase catalyses the formation of carbonic acid (160 mmol/day), and 1 in every 1000 molecules of carbonic acid ionize to form free hydrogen and bicarbonate ions.

$$\frac{H_2CO_3}{H^+HCO_3^-} = \frac{1000}{1} \quad \text{and} \quad \frac{CO_2}{H^+ + HCO_3^-} = \frac{800\,000}{1}.$$

There are 20 molecules of bicarbonate to each molecule of carbonic acid.

$$\frac{HCO_3^-}{CO_2 + H_2CO_3} = \frac{20}{1}.$$

Hydrogen ions attach to basic groups on the haemoglobin molecule, and bicarbonate ions diffuse back into the plasma in exchange for chloride ions entering the cells. Reduced haemoglobin can buffer 27·5 mmol of hydrogen ions per litre, and plasma protein can buffer 4·2 mmol of hydrogen ions per litre. Some carbon dioxide reacts directly with amino acid residues in haemoglobin to form carbamino compounds. In the tissues, as carbon dioxide enters the blood, the plasma pH falls from 7·40 to 7·36 normally.

In the lungs the process is reversed. The high oxygen tension in the alveoli reduces the affinity of the basic groups in haemoglobin for hydrogen ions, and carbon dioxide is regenerated to be expired. The alveolar carbon dioxide tension is roughly equal to the arterial Pa_{CO_2}. In steady state the rate of carbon dioxide excretion equals its rate of formation. The body 'pool' of carbon dioxide is approximately 120 litres, whereas the body 'pool' of oxygen at any moment is only 1 litre.

The body's chemoreceptors can detect changes of 0·1–0·3 kPa (1–2 mmHg) in the Pa_{CO_2} and an increase of this degree above the resting level results in a doubling of the work output of the inspiratory muscles. By contrast the hypoxic ventilatory drive is less sensitive.

There is no significant ventilatory stimulation until the Pa_{O_2} falls to 8 kPa (60 mmHg). The hypoxic and hypercapnoeic drives are synergistic in increasing the depth and then the rate of ventilation. When the carbon dioxide in solution exceeds 6·75–7·43 kPa (50–55 mmHg) high carbon dioxide concentrations act as a narcotic on the respiratory centre in the medulla, the hypoxic drive continuing to stimulate respiration. Carbon dioxide is a cerebral vasodilator, ensuring adequate oxygenation of the brain, but high concentrations can cause cerebral oedema.

$$Normal\ plasma\ Pa_{CO_2} = 5\cdot4\,kPa\ (4\cdot73\text{–}6\cdot08\,kPa)$$
$$or\ 40\,mmHg\ (35\text{–}45\,mmHg).$$

For each rise in Pa_{CO_2} of 1·35 kPa (10 mmHg) the plasma bicarbonate rises by approximately 1 mmol/l, and the ratio of Pa_{CO_2} to HCO_3^- determines the plasma hydrogen ion concentration.

The Pa_{CO_2} is directly proportional to $(CO_{2(d)} + H_2CO_3)$ where the $CO_{2(d)}$ is the dissolved carbon dioxide.

The dissolved $CO_2 = 40 \times 0\cdot03$ mmol/l or $0\cdot226 \times Pa_{CO_2}$ in kPa, where the solubility of carbon dioxide in water $= 0\cdot226$ mmol/l/kPa partial pressure, or 0·03 mmol/l/mmHg partial pressure.

The arterial Pa_{CO_2} is a balance of: (1) rate of production of carbon dioxide; (2) rate of alveolar ventilation. The Pa_{CO_2} has a trivial effect on dissolved carbon dioxide, which is less than 1 mmol/l. Respiratory depression leads to an increase in Pa_{CO_2}. Carbon dioxide diffuses rapidly into the CSF. In the CSF, carbon dioxide in solution stimulates the medullary respiratory centre. The respiratory centres respond to the dominant stimulation of hydrogen ion concentration and P_{CO_2} in the CSF. The peripheral chemoreceptors (cartoid and aortic bodies) with a very large blood flow through them, are very sensitive to depression in the Pa_{CO_2}. A rise in P_{CO_2} from 5·7 to 6·7 kPa (40–50 mmHg) stimulates the respiratory rate fourfold.

Changes in the Pa_{CO_2}

Primary increase in Pa_{CO_2} = respiratory acidosis.
Secondary (compensatory) increase in Pa_{CO_2} = metabolic alkalosis.

Cerebrospinal Fluid and the Brain

Carbon dioxide diffuses freely into cells and into the CSF. Bicarbonate ions diffuse across cell membranes much more slowly. Following increase in Pa_{CO_2} the CSF P_{CO_2} rises, but to a lesser degree. After 1 h the CSF bicarbonate gradually rises, and the CSF hydrogen ion concentration falls towards normal. Carbonic acid, and hence bicarbonate ion, is formed at the choroid plexus to enter the CSF (the reaction being catalysed by carbonic anhydrase). The brain also generates bicarbonate independently of carbonic anhydrase activity. The P_{CO_2} acts on the medullary centre, stimulating respiration, unless the P_{CO_2} exceeds 7·43 kPa (55 mmHg) when carbon dioxide depresses respiratory centre activity.

Pulmonary ventilation is increased fourfold when the CSF pH falls to 7·2, while at pH 7·0 (100 nmol/l) the pulmonary ventilation rate increases eightfold. The depth of respiration increases before the rate increases, and excess carbon dioxide is exhaled.

Depression of the central nervous system is related to carbon dioxide narcosis and also to the CSF pH, and is more profound in respiratory acidosis than in metabolic acidosis (since carbon dioxide is able to diffuse freely across membranes and in and out of cells, while hydrogen ions and bicarbonate ions take hours to equilibrate across cell membranes). In metabolic acidosis the CSF pH is buffered more effectively. The brain pH rises initially in respiratory alkalosis, but then almost immediately there is a fall in bicarbonate concentration and a rise in lactate, which also occurs in the CSF.

Increased Carbon Dioxide ($P_{a CO_2}$)

Signs and Symptoms

1. Loss of appetite, nausea.
2. Headache, lethargy and irritability.
3. Somnolence and confusion.
4. Abnormal EEG readings.
5. Tremors, jerks and clonic movements.
6. CSF pressure often increased.
7. Skin warm and flushed with peripheral vasodilatation.
8. With rapid fall in plasma pH and rise in $P_{a CO_2}$:
   a Heart rate increased.
   b Arrhythmias may develop.
   c Later, as pH approaches 6·8 with rising $P_{a CO_2}$:
       i   Heart rate slows.
       ii Cardiac output reduced.
       iii Responsiveness to catecholamines reduced.
9. With increased intracellular hydrogen ion concentration, (falling pH) is reduced urinary excretion of bicarbonate, with increased ammonium excretion and loss of chloride.

Decreased $P_{a CO_2}$

After overbreathing with resulting very low $P_{a CO_2}$, there is a short period of apnoea, until the hypoxic drive starts respiration once more.

THE RELATIONSHIP BETWEEN THE Pa_{CO_2} AND Pa_{O_2}

The barometric pressure at sea level = 760 mmHg. This is made up of:

Nitrogen   563 mmHg ⎱ no net movement of these across the
Water vapour   47 mmHg ⎰ alveolar capillary.
Oxygen $\dfrac{150 \text{ mmHg}}{760 \text{ mmHg}}$ (i.e. the partial pressure of oxygen in the inspired air = 150 mmHg).

In the alveolus the inspired oxygen enters the blood to combine with haemoglobin, and carbon dioxide leaves the blood and enters the alveolus. The respiratory quotient on an average normal diet = 0·8, i.e. each molecule of carbon dioxide produced and entering the alveolus results from the utilization of 1·25 molecules of oxygen (4 molecules of carbon dioxide are formed from 5 molecules of oxygen). The partial pressure of alveolar oxygen $(P_{alv}O_2)$ = partial pressure of inspired oxygen $(P_{insp}O_2) - 1·25 \times$ partial pressure of alveolar carbon dioxide $(P_{alv}CO_2)$, i.e.

$$P_{alv}O_2 = P_{insp}O_2 - 1·25\, P_{alv}CO_2.$$

Since carbon dioxide diffuses across the alveolar capillary 20 × faster than oxygen, then:

$$P_{alv}CO_2 = P_{insp}O_2 - 1·25\, Pa_{CO_2}$$
$$= 150 - (1·25 \times 40)$$
$$= 100 \text{ mmHg}.$$

Alveolar oxygen partial pressure = PA_{O_2}
Blood oxygen partial pressure = Pa_{O_2}
Inspired air oxygen partial pressure = P_iO_2.
(Alveolar − arterial oxygen gradient = $PA_{O_2} - Pa_{O_2}$.)

$$Pa_{O_2} = PA_{O_2} - (A-a)\text{oxygen gradient}$$
$$= P_iO_2 - 1·25\, Pa_{CO_2} - (A-a) \text{ oxygen gradient}.$$

The (A − a) oxygen gradient $= P_iO_2 - 1·25\, Pa_{O_2} - Pa_{O_2}$
$= normally\ 10\ mmHg\ or\ less.$

The ventilation rate is stimulated by hypoxaemia when the Pa_{O_2} falls below 60–65 mmHg.

$$Pa_{O_2} = PA_{O_2} - (A-a)_{O_2} \text{ gradient} - 1·25\, Pa_{CO_2}$$

or

$$65 = 150 - 1·25\, Pa_{CO_2} - 10$$

Therefore, when $Pa_{O_2} = 65$ mmHg, $Pa_{CO_2} = \dfrac{(150 - 10 - 65)}{1·25}$

$$= \dfrac{75}{1·25}$$
$$= 60 \text{ mmHg}.$$

During respiratory compensation of metabolic alkalosis, the Pa_{CO_2} rarely rises above 60 mmHg, since increased ventilation lowers it again, unless there is respiratory dysfunction.

The $(A-a)$ oxygen gradient may become increased in chronic obstructive pulmonary disease, but both acute and chronic pulmonary disease need not be associated with carbon dioxide retention.

CEREBROSPINAL FLUID
Sodium

CSF sodium concentration: 123–154 mmol/l. The concentration follows the plasma concentration.

Potassium

CSF potassium concentration approximately 3 mmol/l (2.89 ± 0.26 mmol/l). The CSF concentration, which is independent of the plasma concentration, depends on carrier-mediated transport of potassium across the choroid plexus from plasma to CSF. There is exchange of CSF potassium with brain potassium.

Chloride

CSF chloride concentration: 122–132 mmol/l, with the level higher than in the plasma because of the Donnan equilibrium effect of the plasma proteins.

Calcium

CSF ionized calcium concentration is higher than in the plasma. There is a 5 mV electrochemical gradient between CSF and plasma and there is no simple equilibrium between CSF and plasma calcium concentrations.

P_{CO_2}

The CSF P_{CO_2} is higher than Pa_{CO_2} (e.g. CSF $P_{CO_2}=6.5$ kPa (48 mmHg) when the plasma $Pa_{CO_2}=5.4$ kPa (40 mmHg).

pH

CSF pH is lower than plasma pH, e.g. pH 7.32 when plasma pH $=7.40$.

Bicarbonate

CSF bicarbonate concentration is related to CSF pH and P_{CO_2}. Although carbon dioxide diffuses freely and rapidly across the choroid plexus, neither hydrogen ions nor bicarbonate ions can readily cross the blood–CSF barrier, and equilibration takes hours.

CHLORIDE
Absorption

Normally all the chloride in the diet is absorbed. In the stomach and jejunum the osmotic pressure across the mucous membrane is equalized with that of the plasma. Absorption of chloride in the form of passive transport with active transport of sodium occurs in the small intestine; and in the lower ileum and large intestine there is active absorption, with a chloride/bicarbonate exchange. In cholera and other severe intestinal infections, the chloride/bicarbonate exchange is enhanced, with dangerously excessive loss of sodium bicarbonate in liquid stools.

Function of Chloride

Chloride is the main extracellular anion. The extracellular fluid concentration is approximately 103 mmol/l, while the intracellular fluid chloride concentration is 4 mmol/l. The distribution of chloride across the cell membrane is determined by the electrical potential. The resting membrane potential of neuronal soma = -70 mV, while the resting membrane potential of skeletal muscle fibre = -85 mV. With the development of an action potential, chloride ions move rapidly through the cell membrane and affect the duration and magnitude of the action potential passively. With the return to resting membrane potential, chloride ions move out of the cells again.

Body Distribution
1. Plasma Chloride

Normal concentration = 102 mmol/l (95–105). Plasma from venous blood contains 1·5 per cent less chloride than plasma from arterial blood. Red cell carbonic anhydrase catalyses production of bicarbonate from carbon dioxide in venous blood. Since potassium is held inside the cells and sodium is constantly being pumped out, as bicarbonate diffuses out of the red cells in venous blood, chloride ions diffuse into the red cells—the chloride shift. On oxygenation in the lungs, chloride diffuses out of the cells again, when carbon dioxide is exhaled.

2. Intracellular chloride

Concentration approximately 4 mmol/l, but increased in red cells in venous blood, and in muscle and nerve cells during action potential. The chloride concentration is increased in chloride-secreting cells in:

    a   Gastrointestinal mucosa.
    b   Skin.
    c   Ovaries.
    d   Testes.

The cortical chloride concentration in brain = 35–45 mmol/kg wet weight. Chloride is also present in connective tissue and bone.

3. ISF Chloride

Concentration: 114 mmol/l. *Transudates + oedema fluid*: 123–128 mmol/l.

4. Cerebrospinal Fluid Chloride

Concentration = 123–128 mmol/l (consequence of Donnan equilibrium across the capillary walls of the choroid plexus).

5. Tears

Concentration: 115 mmol/l.

6. Total Exchangeable Chloride

Total exchangeable chloride = 27·8–32·8 mmol/kg (higher in men than women), e.g. approximately 2100 mmol per 70-kg man.

7. Sweat

Sweat chloride concentration can reach up to 60 mmol/l, decreasing with acclimatization to heat, when sweating occurs at a lower body temperature than before acclimatization, and the salt content of the sweat is reduced. In trained athletes during strenuous exercise, salt secretion is low, but lactic acid concentration in sweat exceeds the concentration in both plasma and urine (specific gravity: 1·002–1·005 with pH 4·5–7·5).

Gastrointestinal Secretion of Chloride

    1. Saliva: 20–40 mmol/l, reaching 1200 mmol/day.
    2. Gastric juice
        a   Gastric mucus—115 mmol/l.

  b Parietal juice—up to 166 mmol/l, reaching 2560–5120 mmol/day.

Chloride ions in the gastric juice in the form of hydrochloric acid, are secreted by active energy-consuming mechanisms. The same 'pump' carries bromide and iodide ions. The potential difference at the gastric mucous membrane is 30–50 mV. A small part of the gastric juice is so-called 'neutral chloride', sodium and potassium chloride.

  3. Jejunum—80 mmol/l } 3080 mmol/day.
    Ileum—105 mmol/l

  4. Bile: 40–80 mmol/l, 1200 mmol/day. (Liver bile 75–110 mmol/l.)

  5. Pancreatic juice: 10–60 mmol/l, 1370 mmol/day. The secreted choride is reabsorbed in the gastrointestinal tract and recycled.

Renal Treatment of Chloride

Glomerular filtrate contains 18 000 mmol/day, and 17 850 mmol are reabsorbed each day, with 150 mmol chloride excreted in the urine each day on an average normal intake.

  There is passive reabsorption of chloride with active sodium reabsorption in the proximal renal tubule, i.e. seven-eighths of the filtrate reabsorbed with water. Sodium reabsorption is linked with secretion of hydrogen ions in the proximal and distal renal tubules. In the ascending thick limb of the loop of Henle there is active reabsorption of chloride with passive reabsorption of sodium. Aldosterone stimulation results in almost complete reabsorption of sodium and chloride in the distal renal tubules from the luminal fluid. Chloride reabsorption increases as bicarbonate reabsorption decreases, and vice versa. Within 2 weeks of fasting, the urine chloride output falls to 5 mmol/day.

Urine Chloride

Normal 24-h output = dietary intake = 110–225 mmol/day. Normal renal threshold for chloride is thought to be about 96 mmol/l. There is a marked diurnal variation in chloride excretion, with urinary chloride excretion during sleep falling to one-fifth of the excretion rate during the day.

  Following a chloride load, the excess is eliminated over a 48-h period. Following chloride depletion, the urinary chloride falls to very low levels over a 48-h period. After trauma and/or surgery, there is retention of sodium, chloride and water, and at this time absence of chloride from the urine does not necessarily indicate chloride deficiency.

Raised Plasma Chloride

Pure dehydration.

Excessive saline infusion with water loss (e.g. excess 'physiological' saline)

Renal disease.

Diabetes mellitus during treatment of ketoacidosis.

Hyperchloraemic acidosis.

Respiratory alkalosis from prolonged assisted ventilation.

Relatively greater loss of sodium to chloride

Diarrhoea.

Intestinal fistula.

Increased reabsorption of chloride

Ureterocolic anastomosis.

Diuretics

Acetazolamide.

Thiazides (relatively greater loss of sodium than chloride).

Primary hyperparathyroidism (plasma bicarbonate falls with rising chloride).

Cortisol ⎫
Aldosterone ⎬ retention of chloride with sodium.

Ammonium chloride load

Reduced Plasma Chloride

Low salt intake.

Gastric hydrochloric acid loss (i.e. greater loss of chloride than sodium)

Vomiting.

Pyloric stenosis.

Untreated diabetic ketoacidosis.

Potassium depletion.

Excessive sweating in hot climate before acclimatization.

Renal chloride loss

RTA.

Addison's disease.

Mercurial diuretics (greater loss of chloride relative to sodium).

Excess bicarbonate therapy (e.g. post cardiac arrest).

(Acute porphyria).

Paracentesis—rapid removal of salt-containing ascitic fluid.

Increased body water content, e.g. SIADH.

Chronic chloride depletion described in infants fed on soy meal feed with low chloride content.

Congenital chloride loser [R]—stools contain excess chloride, there is consequently bicarbonate generation with potassium loss, leading to hypokalaemic alkalosis, responding to 3–5 mmol potassium chloride/kg body weight/day.

Signs and Symptoms of Chloride Depletion

Weakness and lethargy with severe hypokalaemic alkalosis. Erythrocyturia described in chloride-depleted infants.

CORTISOL
Synthesis

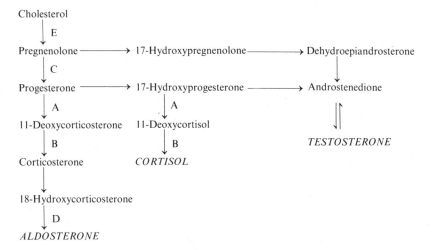

ACTH is secreted episodically in bursts. These result in increased adrenal blood flow and a fall in lipid and ascorbic acid in fascicular cells. These cells are transferred into 'compact' reticular zone cells; 10 min after ACTH, cortisol is secreted, especially in the morning and least frequently for a few hours prior to sleep. Secretion of ACTH decreases within 2 min of a rise in plasma cortisol. A sustained high plasma cortisol level suppresses ACTH release, and a low plasma cortisol level stimulates ACTH release (and hence cortisol release) via CRF (corticotrophin release factor).

Normal Plasma Cortisol

08.00 hrs—280–690 nmol/l.
Midnight—55–280 nmol/l.

There is a circadian rhythm varying with sleeping and waking pattern, with a peak at about 08.00 hrs, falling through the day, with possibly smaller peaks at 12 noon and again at about 18.00 hrs. Lowest levels are reached by midnight. This periodicity is established by 3 years.

Cortisol is normally 80 per cent bound to alpha-globulin, transcortin binding sites, with some binding to albumin, and about 10 per cent free—the free cortisol is thought to be the active portion. Transcortin binding sites are saturated when plasma cortisol levels exceed 280 nmol/l. Plasma cortisol has a biological half-life of 70–80 min. Corticosterone, with a qualitatively similar activity to cortisol, is secreted at one-tenth the rate of cortisol. Cortisone is biologically inert, and has to be converted in the body to cortisol, before it becomes active.

Actions

Cortisol inhibits RNA and DNA synthesis in lymphoid and connective tissue. It stimulates RNA and DNA synthesis in liver and other viscera. In normal pregnancy cortisol may help to mobilize free amino acids for uptake by the growing fetus, for tissue synthesis.

Cortisol facilitates the actions of glucagon, adrenaline and human growth hormone, by inhibition of peripheral glucose utilization. It exerts a so-called 'ketogenic effect' by its synergistic effect on lipolysis in adipose tissue. Protein synthesis is reduced and there is an increase in free amino acids available for gluconeogenesis. Following increased insulin secretion, which, in turn, is in response to the rise in blood glucose, liver glycogen synthetase is activated, with increased liver glycogen synthesis. Thus, gluconeogenesis is maintained by provision of free amino acids (some from peripheral muscle), and by enzyme induction, resulting in a slow body defence against hypoglycaemia. In addition, cortisol is anti-inflammatory and anti-allergic. It increases the RPF, GFR and free water clearance by the kidney, and acts on the distal renal tubule to promote sodium and water retention. The net renal effect is the maintenance of the ability to excrete a water load efficiently. The peripheral arteriolar response to vasoconstrictors is potentiated and permeability of vascular endothelium is reduced.

Cortisol plays an important part in maturation of the fetal lung, and the ability to secrete surfactant.

Pharmacology

Cortisol is used in replacement therapy of both primary and secondary adrenocortical insufficiency. It is also used in the treatment of shock:
1   To increase heart strength.
2   To decrease intracellular lysosomal release.
3   To aid glucose metabolism in severely damaged cells (?).

Pathology
1. *Cortisol Deficiency*
Signs and Symptoms
There is anorexia with weight loss, weakness and apathy. There is also inability to withstand 'stress'. Plasma sodium concentration falls, and plasma potassium and magnesium levels rise with reduced GFR if there is salt restriction. Urine sodium output is inappropriately high, with reference to the plasma sodium concentration, and the urine potassium output is low. In crisis, there is gross salt depletion, hypotension, increased cell potassium, cell hypoxia and oliguria.

Causes
a Primary adrenocortical insufficiency.
b Secondary adrenocortical insufficiency.
c Sudden cessation of prolonged treatment with corticosteroids or ACTH.
d Congenital adrenal hyperplasia (with excess androgens).

A. **21-*Alpha-hydroxylase Deficiency***
Ninety-five per cent of all cases of congenital adrenal hyperplasia. There is impairment of synthesis of both cortisol and aldosterone, with raised plasma ACTH levels. Mild form: virilization in females, pseudo-precocious puberty in males. Severe form (33 per cent of cases): excessive loss of sodium in urine, with low plasma sodium, raised plasma potassium plus metabolic acidosis.

B. **11-*Beta-hydroxylase Deficiency***
The next most frequent variety of congenital adrenal hyperplasia. There is impairment of synthesis of cortisol and corticosterone. Infants suffer from hypertension and virilization. Secondary increase in production of deoxycortisone (DOC) occurs, with signs and symptoms of mineralocorticoid excess. The high plasma ACTH levels stimulate androgen production. (C, D and E are rare enzyme deficiencies.)

2. *Cortisol Excess*
Signs and Symptoms
Hyperglycaemia, diabetes mellitus, excess water and sodium retention, and negative nitrogen balance occur. There is retardation of growth, wasting of muscles, thinning of the skin, osteoporosis and reduction in lymphoid tissue.

Redistribution of body fat occurs, with increased trunk deposition at the expense of peripheral deposits. Muscle weakness is present, following loss of muscle protein and creatine. The patient may suffer from euphoria, restlessness and excitement. Increased gastric acidity is present, and blood lipids increase with atherosclerotic changes.

Causes (preceded by loss of diurnal rhythm)
a   Cushing's syndrome.
b   Prolonged high dosage of glucocorticoids.
c   Hypothyroidism.
d   Hypothermia.
e   Liver disease.
f   Terminal states.
g   Unbalanced diabetes mellitus.

Excretion of Cortisol

Cortisol is metabolized in the liver and conjugated with glucuronic acid to form water-soluble substances, which are excreted in the urine. Estimation of urinary output of cortisol metabolites depends on the method used:

Normal (fluorimetry)—adult males: 210–1100 nmol/24 h—adult females: 210–800 nmol/24 h.

Normal (RIA)—adult males: 350 nmol/24 h—adult females: 290 nmol/24 h.

Urine Output of Cortisol Derivatives Increased

1   Cushing's syndrome
2   Obesity
3   Hirsute female   } suppressed by low-dose
4   Severely depressed patient   dexamethasone test.
5   Alcoholics

Urine 17-oxogenic steroids give a measure of excretion of cortisol metabolite excretion.

CREATININE

Source

Exogenous

Creatinine occurs in the outer surfaces of roast and well-grilled meats. It is the anhydride of creatine.

Endogenous

Creatine is synthesized in the liver, enters the blood, and is taken up by muscle. In the muscle it is converted to creatine phosphate, a high-energy compound, in the resting state. Some of the body store of creatine is lost by a slow transformation to creatinine, which enters the blood, and is excreted in the urine.

Creatine occurs predominantly in skeletal muscle, but is also in cardiac muscle, the muscle of the uterus, especially in pregnancy, and in the brain.

Normal Plasma Creatinine

80–150 μmol/l (0·9–1·7 mg/100 ml).

Increased Plasma Creatinine

1   Dietary increase (roast meats, etc.).
2   Falling GFR—renal damage.

Decrease in Plasma Creatinine

Loss of muscle mass. The plasma concentration is already low, and estimation is not able to detect significant falls in plasma creatinine.

Normal CSF Creatinine

40–135 μmol/l (0·45–1·5 mg/100 ml).

Normal Urine Creatinine Output

Adult male: 13·2–17·6 mmol/day (1·5–2·0 g/day).
Adult female: 7·04–13·2 mmol/day (0·8–1·5 g/day).
Plasma creatinine concentration begins to rise above normal when the GFR falls below 30 ml/min.

Renal Excretion of Creatinine

Creatinine is filtered almost completely by the glomeruli and tubular excretion of creatinine occurs with normal renal function, if exogenous creatinine is given. The urinary output of creatinine increases during muscular work, to be followed by very low urinary creatinine output afterwards at rest.

On average over periods of days, the day-to-day excretion of creatinine in an individual is constant, and directly related to the body muscle mass. The creatinine clearance is 75–125 per cent of the corresponding inulin clearance, and is not affected by decrease in urine flow rate, or by protein intake in the diet (cf. urea). The creatinine clearance tends to the greater than the inulin clearance in renal damage because some creatinine is excreted by the tubules.

Increased Creatinine Output in Urine

1 Acromegaly.
2 Gigantism.
3 Hypothyroidism.
4 Infections.
5 Diabetes mellitus.

Decreased Creatinine Output in the Urine

1 Hyperthyroidism.
2 Muscle disease.
3 Advanced renal disease.
4 Following exposure to heat. It appears that some chromogens measured during the estimation of creatine are lost in the sweat.
5 Bypass operation for adiposity. The lean body muscle mass decreases.

Increased or decreased creatinine outputs are of very little clinical value.

Creatinine clearance is estimated to give a rough indication of the true GFR. Because of its constant output, 24-h urine creatinine is used to compare other solute excretion rates, and to determine that 24-h urine collection is accurate.

Amniotic Fluid

The normal fetus excretes urea and creatinine and other nitrogenous waste into the amniotic fluid. Creatinine is detectable in the amniotic fluid by the twentieth week, and creatinine concentration rises progressively until term. The creatinine concentration can be used to give an approximate estimate of fetal maturity, to within 4 weeks.

GLUCOSE
Normal Plasma Glucose

Whole blood glucose = plasma glucose $\times (1 - (0.3 \times \text{haematocrit}))$.

Concentration of glucose in serum or plasma (if fresh, or glucose preserved), is approximately 14 per cent higher than in whole blood.

Red blood cells and liver cells contain a little free glucose which is freely exchangeable with the ECF. Glucose normally flows out of the ECF pool into the peripheral tissues, but in the fasting state glucose uptake by tissues other than the brain is very low. After food intake there is rapid peripheral tissue uptake of glucose— the arterial and capillary blood glucose concentrations exceeding that of the corresponding venous blood by up to 1·8 mmol/l (40 mg/100 ml). At any one time the glucose in the ECF in the normal adult is up to 20 g.

The liver stores glucose as glycogen, which is synthesized from glucose, and which may also be synthesized from lactate, pyruvate, glycerol or amino acids. After an overnight fast, if the plasma glucose is less than 3 mmol/l or more than 6 mmol/l further investigations are indicated. The glucose present in plasma separated rapidly after collection is relatively stable. The glucose in blood samples preserved with fluoride is stable.

In the presence of a sustained hyperglycaemia, plasma sodium falls by 2·8 mmol/l for each rise of 5·6 mmol/l (100 mg/dl) in blood glucose.

CSF Glucose

CSF glucose concentration is approximately 0·6 times the corresponding plasma glucose concentration in the absence of disease.

HYDROGEN ION CONCENTRATION (pH)

$$pH = -\log\left(\frac{1}{H^+}\right) \quad \text{(as mol/l)}$$

Thus, pH 7·0 = hydrogen ion concentration of 10^2 nmol/l, since:

$$\text{antilog } (H^+) = 10^{-7} \text{ mol/l hydrogen ions}$$
$$= 10^{-7} \times 10^9 \text{ nmol/l}$$
$$= 10^2 \text{ nmol/l}$$

Or another example, using the normal body pH of 7·4:

$$pH \ 7·4 = 9 - 1·6$$
$$\text{antilog } pH = -10^{-9} \times \text{antilog } 1·6$$
$$= 10^{-9} \times 40 \text{ mol/l}$$
$$= 40 \text{ nmol/l}$$
$$40 \text{ nmol/l} = 40 \times 10^{-9} \text{ mol/l}$$
$$pH = -(\log 40 + 10^{-9})$$
$$= -\log 40 - \log 10^{-9}$$
$$= -1·6 - (-9)$$
$$= -1·6 + 9$$
$$= 7·4$$

Normal Plasma pH = 7·35–7·45 (7·40)
Normal Plasma Hydrogen Ion Concentration = 45–35 nmol/l (40)
Venous blood = 40–46 nmol/l
Arterial blood = 37–42 nmol/l
Extreme ranges compatible with life
pH 6·9–7·7 (or 120–20 nmol/l) or possibly 6·8–7·8 (158–16 nmol/l)
Urine pH range
pH 4·5–7·8 or 40 000 nmol/l–16 nmol/l.
Gastric acidity rises to 100 mmol/l (pH 1·0).
Cerebrospinal fluid pH is maintained at 7·3 (50 nmol/l). Free hydrogen ions act on chemoreceptors in the medulla oblongata.

Body Metabolism

During cell metabolism, protein, fat and carbohydrate catabolism, hydrogen ions are liberated at the rate of 60 mmol/day (50–100 mmol/day) or 60 000 nmol/day or approximately 1 mmol/kg body weight per day.

The ECF contains 40 nmol/l × 15 litre = 600 nmol.

Renal maximum excretion rate = 600 mmol hydrogen ions per day or approximately 0·3 mmol hydrogen ions per minute. With no ventilation (respiration) hydrogen ions accumulate at the rate of 10 mmol/min. Ventilation (respiration) enables hydrogen ions to be excreted:

$$H^+ + HCO_3^- \rightleftharpoons H_2CO_3 \rightleftharpoons H_2O + CO_2.$$

$[H^+]$ depends on ratio of PCO_2 to $[HCO_3]$.

Renal Excretion

(Titratable acid + ammonium excretion) in urine = bicarbonate regenerated by renal tubules.

Normal

Of renal hydrogen ion excretion 97–98 per cent is consumed by renal luminal bicarbonate.

Two to three per cent of renal hydrogen ion excretion is as titratable acid.

Ammonia production (and hence urine ammonium) governs the final urine pH.

Normal urine pH averages 6·0, as more hydrogen ion is excreted than bicarbonate ion. Fifty to one hundred mmol H^+ in the form of non-volatile acid (sulphuric and phosphoric acids) are produced each day from catabolism of protein, and 50–100 mmol HCO_3^- are regenerated in renal tubules each day.

The net hydrogen ion excretion in the urine = (titratable acid + ammonium excretion) − (bicarbonate excretion).

Increased Plasma Hydrogen Ion Concentration (falling pH)

1. Increased Production

Diabetic keto-acidosis

Cellular anoxia—with production of lactic acid, etc.

2. Buffer Loss

Gastrointestinal fluid loss
Small bowel fluid loss
Pancreatic fluid loss
Biliary fluid loss

3. Decreased Hydrogen Ion Excretion

Kidney damage
Bicarbonate exchange defect
Ammonia synthesis defect
Respiratory damage
Reduced alveolar ventilation with reduction in carbon dioxide excretion

INTERSTITIAL FLUID (ISF)

The interstitial fluid makes up 15–25 per cent of the total body weight (varying from up to 70 per cent in loose connective tissue to 10 per cent in skeletal muscle).

Function

It acts as a transport medium for nutrients and waste products. It also acts as a buffer fluid volume for plasma and neighbouring cells, until other mechanisms adjust fluid balance towards normal.

Structure

The normal interstitium consists of glycosaminoglycan-containing gel-like matrix embedded in a network of collagen fibres. In consequence the ISF has greatly restricted mobility.

Regulation

It appears that the ISF is self-adjusting, with structural resistance aganist volume change, self-adjustment of the Starling forces, including local vasomotor reactions, and automatic adjustment of lymph flow according to local needs.

There is resistance to the transfer of fluid from plasma in hypervolaemia (i.e. resistance to oedema formation), and resistance to transfer of fluid from the ISF to plasma in hypovolaemia (i.e. resistance to interstitial fluid dehydration). Changes in plasma volume, and effective circulating volume therefore trigger reactions sooner rather than later.

LACTIC ACIDOSIS

Energy Requirements in the Body

1. Brain

The brain has a constant energy requirement, unaffected by exertion or sleep, amounting to 25 per cent of the total energy requirement of the resting adult. This is met by 120 g glucose daily, which is catabolized to carbon dioxide and water, with energy release.

2. Red and White Blood Cells

Red cells and white cells have no mitochondria, and therefore are obligatory lactic acid producers. They convert the equivalent of 36 g glucose to lactate each day, and this is taken from the blood by the liver and metabolized.

3. Resting Body

The normal man produces 25–30 mmol/kg body weight of lactic acid each day. The extrahepatic tissues produce more lactate than can be catabolized by reactions other than the conversion of lactate back to pyruvate via lactate dehydrogenase activity. In the tissue cells $(NADH + NAD^+)$ exists predominantly in the NAD^+ form, whereas $(NADPH + NADP^+)$ exists predominantly in the NADPH form. NAD is 100 times as effective as NADP as coenzyme of lactate dehydrogenase (except in the liver, where the two coenzymes act with equal facility).

4. Liver

The main source of energy for liver cells appears to be from amino acids. During starvation energy is derived from the oxidation of fatty acids and glycerol. The liver takes up lactate from the blood and

converts it to pyruvate. Pyruvate can then enter the Krebs citric acid cycle or take part in the formation of fatty acids. During fasting the liver can utilize amino acids to form glucose. The liver can store up to 90 g of glycogen, derived from carbohydrate absorbed in the food. Liver glycogen can be formed from:
  a. Hexose monosaccharide in the food.
  b. Intermediate carbohydrate catabolism products, e.g. lactate, pyruvate.
  c. Glycerol following the hydrolysis of fat.
  d. Amino acid metabolism.

The major part of the lactate produced during exercise is taken up by the liver and metabolized. During very strenuous exercise, plasma lactate levels rise, with falling plasma bicarbonate, pH and increasing 'oxygen debt'. Oxidation of fat, as occurs in starvation, results in increased production of NADH at the expense of NAD^+ (this also occurs in alcohol poisoning). Lactic acid estimations are not useful as a test of liver damage.

5. Kidney

Kidney is able to convert lactate to pyruvate, and can form glucose from amino acids, but not to the same degree as the liver.

6. Muscle

a. Muscle at Rest

Probably the main energy source for resting muscle is fat oxidation, with less than 30 g glucose needed each day.

b. Mild Exertion

There is increased oxidation of fatty acids and their derivatives, with no increase in blood lactate.

c. Vigorous Exercise

The blood supply to the muscles is greatly increased, as the muscle mechanical output can increase 64-fold. There is a switch to carbohydrate catabolism, and the lactic acid content of venous blood draining active muscle is greater than the lactate equivalent of glucose uptake by the muscles, i.e. muscle glycogen is being broken down. When muscle glycogen is used up in severe prolonged exercise, the blood glucose concentration falls markedly, and this coincides with a feeling of severe fatigue. The muscle continues with high energy output using fatty acids once more. More ATP is generated during glucose catabolism than during fat catabolism, and the generation of sufficient ATP is vital for muscle contraction, but ATP is generated at the expense of the generation of hydrogen ions during anaerobic glycolysis. Thus, lactic acid and hydrogen ion concentrations increase during severe exercise.

Anaerobic Glycolysis

The intermediate product of glucose catabolism is pyruvate (Reaction 1).

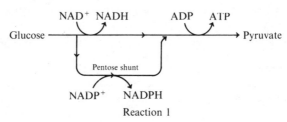

Reaction 1

If oxygen is freely available then pyruvate can:

a. Undergo oxidative decarboxylation of acetylcoenzyme A, as an initial stage before either oxidation to carbon dioxide and water, with release of ATP, or conversion to fatty acid. (Reaction 2)

b. Carboxylation to oxalo-acetic acid, as an initial stage towards conversion to glucose or glycogen. (Reaction 3)

Reactions (1), (2) and (3) require mitochondrial oxidative processes and a constant supply of NAD. Conversion of pyruvate to lactate via the activity of the enzyme lactate dehydrogenase with NADH as coenzyme, generates a supply of NAD in the peripheral tissues, including muscle, but at the expense of release of free hydrogen ions. (Reaction 4)

$$\text{Pyruvate} + \text{NADH} \xrightleftharpoons[\substack{\text{lactate dehydrogenase} \\ \text{(anaerobic dehydrogenation} \\ \text{i.e. oxidation)}}]{\text{(reduction)}} \text{Lactate} + \text{NAD}^+$$

Reaction 4

Lactic acid is a strong acid, and is therefore almost completely dissociated in the body fluids, being a very poor buffer. The plasma pH therefore falls. The normal lactate/pyruvate ratio in the cell cytosol $= 4$–$10:1$ ($= \text{NADH}/\text{NAD}^+$).

During the normal resting state the venous blood lactate does not exceed $2\,\text{mmol/l}$, and the liver takes out the lactate in the blood for metabolism. In vigorous exercise, rapid catabolism of glucose to pyruvate, with rapid conversion to lactate, permits a temporary oxygen debt to build up, with utilization of circulating glucose and muscle glycogen.

In disease states, for example, cardiac arrest, the tissues use anaerobic catabolism of glucose, and lactate cannot be reconverted to pyruvate. There is severe lactic acidosis, and death in a few minutes unless the heart is started again.

Signs and Symptoms

Signs and symptoms of the primary disorder causing lactic acidosis. Sudden onset of hyperpnoea, with malaise, nausea and weakness. There is a fall in the blood pressure.

Blood tests reveal metabolic acidosis with an abnormally large anion gap.

Normal Plasma Lactate

0·55–1·70 mmol/l (5–15 mg/100 ml) (i.e. less than 2 mmol/l).

Normal Plasma Pyruvate

0·01–0·11 mmol/l (0·12–1 mg/dl).

Increased Plasma Lactate

1. Physiological

Following vigorous muscular exercise the plasma lactate concentration rises up to 11 mmol/l (100 mg/dl).

2. Pathological

  a   Increased production of lactate.
  b   Decreased utilization of lactate.
  c   (a) and (b) combined.

....

Lactic acidosis Type A = associated with obvious tissue anoxia.
Lactic acidosis Type B = no clinically obvious tissue anoxia.

....

Specific Causes

  a   Traumatic shock.
  b   Cardiac arrest.
  c   Congestive cardiac failure plus exertion.
  d   Liver failure.

e   Pulmonary embolism, pulmonary oedema, causing congestive failure.
f   Asphyxia.
g   Hypoxia.
n   Sepsis.
i   Diabetic ketoacidosis.
j   Severe anaemia.
k   Drugs and toxins
   i   Salicylate poisoning.
   ii   Phenformin and biguanides in treatment of diabetes mellitus.
   iii   Methanol poisoning.
   iv   Ethanol excess. Alcohol conversion to acetate involves use of NAD and generation of NADH plus free hydrogen ions.
   v   Ethylene glycol poisoning.
   vi   Paraldehyde excess.
   vii   Cyanide poisoning.
l   'Idiopathic' lactic acidosis.
m   Hereditary lactic acidosis
   i   Glucose-6-phosphatase deficiency.
   ii   Fructose-1,6-diphosphatase deficiency.
   iii   Pyruvate carboxylase deficiency.
   iv   Pyruvate dehydrogenase deficiency.
   v   Defects in oxidative phosphorylation.
   vi   Subacute necrotizing encephalomyelitis of Leigh.

Treatment

1. Treat the cause.
2. Infusion of intravenous sodium bicarbonate solution at the rate of up to 300–500 mmol during the first few hours, with diuretics, if renal function is satisfactory.

MAGNESIUM

Dietary Intake

In Northern Europe the dietary intake from green vegetables and meat from an average diet is 10–20 mmol/l (20–40 mEq/day).

Absorption

Of the dietary magnesium 30–40 per cent is absorbed in the small intestine. Since magnesium absorption is enhanced by the presence of protein, magnesium supplements should be given as magnesium salts with food. When magnesium salts are given without food, they tend to cause diarrhoea. Vitamin D plays a small part in the absorption of magnesium. A high intake of fat, phosphate, calcium or alkalis interferes with magnesium absorption. Magnesium is absorbed from the small intestine in renal failure, whereas calcium absorption is impaired. On a diet with a low magnesium content, 75 per cent of the magnesium is absorbed, whereas on a high magnesium diet only 25 per cent is absorbed.

Function

Magnesium plays an important part in bone structure. It is involved in cell permeability regulation, and neuromuscular excitability. It is a co-factor for many enzyme systems, including ATPase, and is involved in DNA function.

Distribution

Fifty per cent of the total body magnesium is in the ICF (500 mmol). Approximately 50 per cent of the total body magnesium is in the bones, and 30 per cent of this is readily exchangeable. One-third of the total body magnesium is exchangeable.

Two per cent of the body magnesium is in the ECF—32 per cent bound to protein, 13 per cent complement to non-protein anion, 55 per cent ionized.

Twenty per cent of the body magnesium is in the muscle.

Erythrocyte magnesium estimation gives a measure of intracellular magnesium levels (the concentration is 50 per cent higher in reticulocytes).

Plasma Magnesium

0·75–1 mmol/l (1·5–2 mEq/l). The range compatible with life = 0·5–3 mmol/l (1–6 mEq/l). Plasma protein-bound magnesium varies from 20 to 30 per cent, with the unbound, mostly ionized, portion 80–70 per cent.

Faecal Excretion

The faeces contain 40–70 per cent of the dietary magnesium—approximately 6 mmol/day.

Urine Excretion

The urinary output of magnesium represents 30–60 per cent of the dietary intake, approximately 4 mmol/day, which represents 8–10 per cent of the glomerular filtrate; 25 per cent of the magnesium in the glomerular filtrate is reabsorbed in the proximal renal tubule and 60–70 per cent is reabsorbed in the ascending loop of Henle and the distal tubule. The proportion reabsorbed is regulated by the plasma magnesium concentration. The possible urinary magnesium range is 0·5–250 mmol/day.

The glomerular filtrate contains 70–80 per cent of the plasma magnesium filtered, i.e. the non-protein-bound portion.

On a magnesium-free diet normal subjects excrete 0·5 mmol magnesium per day.

1. *Increased Urine Magnesium Excretion*

  a Diuretic action
       Ethacrynic acid.
       Frusemide.
       Thiazides.
       Mercurial diuretics.
  b Hypercalcaemia with hypercalciuria.
  c Chronic alcoholism.
  d Hyperaldosteronism
       Primary—increased urinary and faecal magnesium.
       Secondary.
  e Hyperthyroidism.
  f Chronic renal failure.
  g Diabetic ketoacidosis. There is loss of magnesium with ketoacids.
  h Renal tubular acidosis.
  i Gentamicin toxicity.
  j Calcitonin therapy
       In the treatment of hypercalcaemia.
       Paget's disease of bone.
  k Severe hypoparathyroidism. Urine magnesium excretion is increased parallel with the fall in tubular reabsorption of phosphate.

2. *Decreased Urine Magnesium Excretion*

  a Very low dietary magnesium intake.
  b Low magnesium output in some persistent renal stone-formers. The magnesium : calcium ratio is low.

1. *Increased Plasma Magnesium Concentration*
Signs and Symptoms
Ventricular fibrillation develops.

Causes

a Renal insufficiency.
b Adrenal insufficiency rarely.
c Intravenous magnesium salt load followed by hypercalciuria.

Treatment

Ten ml of calcium gluconate are injected slowly intravenously.

2. Decreased Plasma Magnesium Concentration

Signs and Symptoms

a Weakness.
b Tremor.
c Muscles
    Hyperreactive deep reflexes.
    Increased muscle irritability.
    Fibrillation and fasciculation.
    Tetany, positive Chvostek's sign.
d Convulsions.
e Vomiting.
f Ileus.
g Anxiety, disorientation, occasionally psychosis, delirium.
h Blood pressure falls, especially if plasma magnesium falls below
    $0.25\,mmol/l$ (i.e. dangerously low level).
i Positive response to magnesium salt therapy.
j Non-specific ECG changes
    Nodal or sinus tachycardia.
    Inverted T waves.
    ST depression.
k The sensitivity to digitalis glycosides is increased, with increased
    liability to toxicity. Digitalis glycosides reduce the renal tubular
    reabsorption of magnesium, causing progressive deterioration of
    magnesium depletion.

Causes

a Diuretic action.
b Malnutrition.
c Malabsorption.
d Excessive gastrointestinal loss.
e Alcoholism
    i   Often low magnesium intake.
    ii Increased urinary loss due to direct action of alcohol on the
        kidney.

iii Increased faecal magnesium loss.
f Prolonged intravenous fluids/feeding without magnesium supplements.
g Hypokalaemia.
h Hypocalcaemia.
i Severe hypoparathyroidism—plasma magnesium falls following decreased renal tubular reabsorption.

Treatment

a. Twenty-five mmol intravenously over a 6-h period (e.g. 25 ml of 25 per cent magnesium sulphate ($MgSO_4.7H_2O$) solution. Or 0·1 mmol/kg magnesium salt every 6 h intravenously or intramuscularly. If given intravenously, the magnesium solution must be diluted to avoid causing hypotension.

b. Oral magnesium oxide, 6·25–12·5 mmol/day (250–500 mg). This must be given with food to reduce the tendency to produce diarrhoea.

ONCOTIC PRESSURE/COLLOID OSMOTIC PRESSURE
Plasma–ISF Exchange

The equivalent of the whole plasma volume escapes from the entire capillary bed into the ISF and back again in less than 1 min.

In active tissues this exchange increases:
1 Due to increase in blood flow to active tissues.
2 Increase in arteriolar pressure increases outflow of fluid into ISF.
3 Capillaries dilate and previously closed capillaries open up. The capillaries become more permeable.
4 Removal of fluid from ISF
   a Some fluid is retained in tissues.
   b Some fluid escapes into the lymphatics.
   c Fluid is lost in glandular secretion.

Plasma Oncotic Pressure (Colloid Osmotic Pressure)

There is good correlation between plasma total protein and colloid osmotic pressure, unless there is a high proportion of protein other than albumin (e.g. monoclonal gammopathy). The osmotic pressure due to 10 g/l albumin = 6 mmHg and the osmotic pressure due to 10 g globulin = 1·5 mmHg.

The normal plasma colloid osmotic pressure is approximately 28–30 mmHg which consists of approximately 19 mmHg due to plasma protein and 9 mmHg due to cations held by the Donnan effect of proteins.

Fasting and dehydration can increase the colloid osmotic pressure by + 3 per cent, while ambulation for 1 h can increase it by + 15 per cent. When taking blood samples for estimation, it is important that the blood is free-flowing, since use of a tourniquet can increase the colloid osmotic pressure by + 15 per cent. There is no simple correlation between the colloid osmotic pressure and the osmolality of the serum.

Interstitial Fluid

The total volume of the ISF is four times the plasma volume, and the total ISF protein content equals that of the total plasma protein. The ISF protein concentration = 20 g/l (approximately), with a much higher proportion of albumin to globulin than in the plasma. Albumin, with a smaller molecule, diffuses into the ISF more freely. There is 140 per cent turnover of albumin from plasma to ISF and back again daily. The oncotic pressure of the ISF = 5 mmHg.

Plasma Colloid Osmotic Pressure and Development of Pulmonary Oedema

It has been claimed that measurement of colloid osmotic pressure may be useful in the prediction and avoidance of pulmonary oedema, especially if the plasma colloid osmotic pressure is below 10·5 mmHg. On the other hand, patients with chronic hypoproteinaemia with a colloid osmotic pressure of less than 10·5 mmHg do not automatically develop pulmonary oedema. Pulmonary oedema can develop with normal colloid osmotic pressure, and develops when:
1. There is a relative increase in capillary pressure compared with ISF pressure.
2. There is reduction in colloid osmotic pressure of capillary plasma when compared with that of the ISF.
The main determinant of development of pulmonary oedema is the difference between colloid osmotic pressure and pulmonary artery wedge pressure. It is not possible to measure either the pressure or the osmotic pressure of the ISF, but it is possible to measure the pulmonary artery wedge pressure and also the colloid osmotic pressure of either peripheral or pulmonary plasma or serum, and it is desirable to measure both the colloid osmotic and the pulmonary artery wedge pressure to calculate the colloid hydrostatic pressure gradient.
Changes in colloid osmotic pressure measurements alone can give warning of incipient pulmonary oedema, if large volumes of non-blood products have been transfused, but the estimation is of limited use, in general.

OSMOLALITY

The human body is maintained in a state of normal hydration and normal tonicity within well-defined limits. Any deviation outside these limits is followed by adjustments via the volume and rate of respiration (rapid change) and of renal excretion of water and solutes, or their retention (less rapid change).

In the normal state, fluid intake, which usually exceeds compulsory fluid loss, plus food intake, with fluid loss via respiratory evaporation, sweating, renal fluid plus solute excretion, and fluid loss in stools, are accompanied by flexible adjustment of renal fluid and solute excretion, maintaining the normal body status quo.

Thirst and hunger enable the normal individual to maintain adequate nutrition and fluid intake. When food and drink is readily available, eating and drinking at regular times is a habit, rather than a response to the stimuli of hunger and thirst.

Chemoreceptors, osmoreceptors and volume sensors in the body detect small changes in chemical concentration, osmolality, blood pressure and effective circulating volume. The responses of these sensors, and the stimuli generated result in changes in respiration and renal excretion, quantity and concentration of sweat, maintaining or restoring normal homeostasis.

Osmoreceptors, Chemoreceptors and Volume Sensors

The supraoptic nuclear region and adjacent regions of the hypothalamus respond to the injection into the carotid artery of hypertonic fluid (especially hypertonic saline, with less response to hypertonic glucose, and no response to hypertonic urea solutions), by release of ADH plus its carrier protein. The effect of ADH release is increased renal water reabsorption, reducing plasma osmolality, and increased (or reducing rate of decrease) circulating blood volume, detectable by arterial baroreceptors and venous low pressure receptors, and hence in suppression of release of further ADH.

The hypothalamic osmoreceptors are affected by increase in plasma osmolality of $+1-2$ per cent, or by a fall in blood pressure exceeding -10 per cent, causing release of ADH and its carrier protein. When 1 per cent of the ICF water enters the ECF, the hypothalamic region near the paraventricular nucleus (caudal to the osmoreceptors) is stimulated, the conscious animal becomes thirsty, and drinks if fluid is available. Direct electrical stimulation of this area results in active drinking in conscious goats in 10–30 sec, while destruction of this same area results in complete loss of thirst. Thirst also develops when the blood volume is decreased by more than 7–10 per cent, overriding the state of osmolality of the body fluids. Angiotensin II is released in response to reduced blood volume, acting on the hypothalamus to increase thirst, and increasing vasoconstriction. Thirst is suppressed by increase in the effective arterial blood volume, and by decrease in fluid osmolality.

Plasma osmolality greater than 292 mmol/kg is the lowest level at which there is invariably a rise in plasma vasopressin and urine concentration in normal adults.

The ventrolateral surfaces of the medulla respond to changes in CO_2 content and/or hydrogen ion concentration in the CSF, by changes in the depth and rate of respiration, affecting blood Pa_{CO_2}, and indirectly affecting the plasma bicarbonate and hydrogen ion concentration.

The *bodies* in the carotid arteries and the arch of the aorta have a very high blood flow rate through them, with a very small difference in Pa_{O_2} before and after passage through their tissues. If the arterial Pa_{O_2} falls, then the bodies respond by stimulating vasoconstriction, increasing the blood pressure, and increasing the respiration rate. Similar changes follow detection of a fall in blood pressure, which results in a fall in Pa_{O_2} in the carotid and aortic bodies, as a result of reduction in blood flow rate through the bodies. Increased Pa_{CO_2} is followed by increased ventilation volume and rate.

The juxtaglomerular apparatus of the kidney also detects chemical changes in the blood and renal tubular fluid, with feedback responses:

1. Increased circulating angiotensin II results in reduced renin secretion.

2. Sodium retention results in increase in ECF volume, which reduces renin secretion.

3. Increase in blood pressure reduces renin secretion.

4. Systemic vasoconstriction, by increasing blood pressure, also reduces renin secretion.

5. Sodium concentration in the plasma has a direct effect on the macula densa cells. Low sodium concentration is associated with increased renin secretion, while hypernatraemia is associated with suppression of renin secretion.

Sodium receptors are also present in the walls of the cerebral ventricles, detecting changes in sodium concentration. Also osmoreceptors detecting changes in plasma osmolality are present in the liver.

Volume Sensors

There are volume sensors in the thorax and kidneys which affect release of renin, secretion of ADH and vessel tone. Plasma volume and ECF volume affect stretch receptors.

1. *Cardiac Atria*

Branching ends of small medullated fibres connect with the vagus nerves. Type A fibres are concentrated at the entrance of the great veins into the atria, and discharge once per cardiac cycle, beginning with atrial systole, i.e. they are on the low-pressure side of the intrathoracic circulation. Activity is not affected by atrial volume.

Type B receptors discharge with atrial filling, and their activity correlates with atrial size.

A decrease in atrial pressure results in reduced sodium excretion, while an increase in atrial pressure results in increased sodium excretion. This response occurs whether the sodium intake is low or high, in spite of adrenalectomy, and in spite of subsequent mineralocorticoid replacement therapy. When the right atrium is distended, plasma renin levels fall and ADH release is not altered; when the left atrium is distended, plasma renin release is not affected and ADH release is suppressed.

2. *Cardiac Ventricles*

Unmyelinated nerve fibres are derived from the right ventricle.

3. *Unmyelinated Juxtapulmonary Capillary Receptors*

These are present in the lung interstitium. They probably detect interstitial oedema before fluid enters the alveoli. Stretch and tension signals travel via the IX and X nerves to the hypothalamus and medulla and result in ADH release, renal sympathetic nerve discharge and altered tone in pre- and postcapillary resistance vessels in the peripheral vascular bed. Intrathoracic pressure increase results in natriuresis and diuresis (e.g. on immersion in water).

4. *Arterial Volume Sensors*

When the carotid baroreceptors are stretched, there follows an increase in sodium excretion in the urine.

5. *Renal Volume Sensors*

Reduced renal perfusion is followed by renin release, which results in angiotensin II, and, hence, aldosterone release and consequent sodium retention. Increased renal perfusion results in natriuresis. A complicated, and as yet unknown, system of sensors and plain muscle responders convert the fluctuating arterial blood supply delivered by the renal arteries (systolic–diastolic pressure) to a constant pressure supply when it reaches the glomerular tufts.

This brief summary of the various receptors affecting respiration and the urine flow indicates the complexity of the ways in which the human body responds to various stimuli. In pathological states it is possible for different responses apparently to be contradictory to one another, e.g. stretch of right atrium with falling blood pressure in rheumatic heart disease.

Definitions

$Osmolarity$ = mosmol/litre of solution.

$Osmolality$ = mosmol/kg(litre) of water, measured by freezing point difference.

Non-ideality of Solutions

Osmolality/solute concentration ratio increases with solute concentration. Molecular shape affects the slope of the plot. The osmolality of protein solution is dependent on hydrogen ion concentration (pH) (the Gibbs–Donnan ionization effect).

There is a difference between osmolality and osmolarity due to changes in solvent volumes with temperature change. At body temperature this difference is not important. Osmotic pressure is a function of the concentration of active chemical components in a solution, i.e. the number of ions and molecules (undissociated). All internal body fluids tend to have an equal osmotic pressure (both ECF and ICF).

Avogadro's Number

Avogadro's number enables definition of 1 mole to contain $6 \cdot 02 \times 10^{23}$ particles in 1 kg of solution, and 1 millimole to contain $6 \cdot 02 \times 10^{20}$ particles in 1 kg of solution.

One mmol can be translated to mosmol in dilute solutions only, as increasing concentration increases the tendency for particles to pair, and to act as one particle.

Osmotic Coefficient

$$\text{Osmotic coefficient} = \frac{\text{Measurable particles}}{\text{Theoretical no. of particles}}$$

At body temperature the plasma osmolality

$$= ((2 \times Na^+) + glucose + urea) \text{ mosmol/kg approx.}$$

$$= ((2 \times Na^+) + glucose + urea) \text{ mmol/l.}$$

Plasma Osmolality

$$= 2 \times Na(mEq/l) + \frac{Glucose\ mg\%}{18} + \frac{Urea\ mg\%}{60} \left(or\ \frac{Nitrogen\ mg\%}{2\cdot 8} \right)$$

When plasma sodium chloride concentration = 150 mmol/l, the calculated osmolality exerted by sodium chloride = 300 mosmol/l, whereas the measured osmolality by freezing point depression = 279 mosmol/l. The theoretical osmolality of plasma = 325 mosmol/kg water = 305 mosmol/l. The actual plasma osmolality as measured = approx. 290 mosmol/kg, since some electrolytes are not completely dissociated, and some substances partially bind to protein.

Colloid osmotic pressure exerted by plasma proteins across semipermeable membranes of living cells, which are impermeable to protein but permeable to water and some electrolytes, is 2 mosmol/kg.

Osmolality = nc = osmol/kg water = osmotic coefficient
where n = number of particles dissolved in 1 kg water;
c = concentration of solution = mol/kg water.

If a molecule dissociated into 2 or 3 particles, then osmolality due to that original particle increases by × 2 or × 3 respectively. Osmolarity refers to concentration per litre of solution.

Plasma osmolarity = approximately 295–3000 mosmol/l

e.g.			
Sodium	140 mmol/l	× 2	280 mosmol/l
Glucose	6 mmol/l		6 mosmol/l
Urea	6 mmol/l		6 mosmol/l
Protein	2 mmol/l		2 mosmol/l
			294 mosmol/l

(Sodium mmol/l × 2 = cations plus balancing anions, e.g. NaCl)

With rapid changes in plasma osmolarity, the red cell MCV (mean cell volume) varies significantly, falling with dehydration and rising with overhydration, in addition to varying with hydrogen ion concentration (pH).

Urea, ethanol, methanol and ethylene glycol are highly permeable substances, crossing semipermeable cell membranes. They therefore exert little 'effective' osmolality in the ECF. As they do diffuse freely across cell membranes, in high concentration, they increase tonicity, e.g. blood alcohol of 150 mg/dl increases plasma osmolality by + 30 mosmol/kg.

Urine osmolality range = 50–1400 mosmol/kg (corresponding to a specific gravity range of 1·001–1·050).

BLOOD OXYGEN (Pao_2)

Haemoglobin carries 1·34 ml oxygen per g (0·3 ml oxygen in solution in each 100 ml plasma).
Arterial blood oxygen content = 18–21 ml oxygen per 100 dl (arterial blood is 98 per cent saturated, while venous blood is 55–71 per cent saturated).

Pao_2 varies in the Normal Subject with Age

Less than 30 years	12·15–13·50 kPa	(90–100 mmHg)	with 95 per
30–40 years	11·48–12·83 kPa	(85–95 mmHg)	cent
40–60 years	10·13–12·15 kPa	(75–90 mmHg)	oxygen
More than 60 years	8·78–10·80 kPa	(65– 80 mmHg)	saturation.

Available oxygen is highest when the haematocrit is about 0·42. As the haematocrit increases above 0·42, whole blood viscosity rises with increasing peripheral resistance and lower cardiac output.

Cyanosis

This is apparent when more than 5 g per 100 ml of reduced haemoglobin (i.e. not oxygenated) is circulating. If the whole blood total haemoglobin concentration is normal, then there is 75 per cent saturation of haemoglobin with oxygen and Pao_2 = 6·75 kPa (50 mmHg).
Reduction of alveolar ventilation by half results in decrease in Pao_2 to 8·1 kPa (60 mmHg) = hypoxaemia. At Pao_2 8 kPa, cerebral blood flow is increased, and is doubled when Pao_2 falls to 4·7 kPa (35 mmHg). Death is inevitable when Pao_2 falls to 2·7 kPa (20 mmHg).
Total 'stored' oxygen in a normal 70-kg man = 1·75 litres (very small, cf. CO_2 'store')
a Lungs—400 ml
b Arterial blood—300 ml
c Venous blood—600 ml
d Muscles and tissues—300 ml
A total of 750 million alveoli are ventilated during respiration at a rate of 5–6 litres of air per minute:
a One-quarter of inspired air is in the 'dead space'.
b Three-quarters of inspired air is in the alveoli.

During voluntary apnoea (breath-holding time $= 30$–50 sec), the alveolar P_{CO_2} rises to 6.08–6.75 kPa (45–50 mmHg), and the normal conscious subject is then forced to take a breath.

Hyperbaric oxygen $= 3$ atmospheres pressure of 100 per cent oxygen. $Pa_{O_2} = 305$ kPa (2260 mmHg). At least 350 ml of oxygen are available to the tissues per minute by transport of oxygen in simple solution in plasma.

Hypoxia

When the Pa_{O_2} falls below 8.78–8.1 kPa (65–60 mmHg) hypoxia stimulates ventilation depth and rate.

Hypocapnoeic alkalosis secondary to dyspnoea, with increased ventilation due to hypoxia, results in cerebral vasoconstriction, which amplifies the pre-existing hypoxia.

Index of Hypoxic Dysfunction

The ability of the retinal rods to adapt to dark is impaired at 11.48 kPa (85 mmHg) (equivalent to flying in an unpressurized aircraft at 10 000 feet).

Normal Oxygen Consumption

A total of 3.5 ml of oxygen per 100 g brain per min, e.g. a 70-kg man requires 250 ml oxygen per min for the brain—20 per cent of the total body requirement for an organ which is 2 per cent of the total body weight.

Causes of Hypoxia

1. *Newborn*

    a Congenital malformations.
    b Idiopathic respiratory distress syndrome.
    c Pneumonia.
    d Recurrent apnoea.

2. *Later*

    a Asthmatic bronchospasm—falling Pa_{O_2} with rising Pa_{CO_2}. If the Pa_{CO_2} starts to fall towards normal without improvement in Pa_{O_2} the condition is dangerous.
    b Pneumonia ⎫
    c Emphysema ⎰ Respiratory damage.
    d Cardiac failure.

e Postoperation in elderly patients. Pao_2 falls after premedication, and also immediately after operation for the first 24 hours.
f Low oxygen content in inspired air.

3. *Hypoxia uncomplicated by Cerebral Ischaemia*
   a Secondary to lung disease
       with ventilation-diffusion defects.
       with ventilation-perfusion defects.
   b Severe anaemia.

PAEDIATRIC PROBLEMS

When compared with an adult, the younger the child the greater are the differences.

1. Premature Infant (compared with adult)

a Relative excess of body water.
b Larger visceral organ mass relative to the total body.
c Smaller relative muscle mass, and therefore a smaller reserve of protein and potassium.
d Greater vulnerability of the pulmonary system.
e Renal immaturity.
f Less effective ventilation and temperature regulation systems.

Premature infant	40% of the body weight = ECF
Fullterm infant	35% of the body weight = ECF
1–4 years old	30% of the body weight = ECF
Adult	16% of the body weight = ECF

2. Normal Birth

Normal birth is followed by a period of rapid growth, during the first 2 years of which the brain is susceptible to damage from anoxia, hypoglycaemia and electrolyte disturbances.

3. Infant

The normal baby has a small mass with a relatively large surface area, and can lose both heat and water rapidly and dangerously by evaporation. An obese baby becomes dehydrated more rapidly than a normal baby.
   The maximum urine concentration is up to 700 mosmol/kg, reaching a ceiling of 1500 mosmol/kg by 1 year. Since the average urine osmolality is 300 osmol/kg, babies can easily be overloaded with fluid.

The obligatory urine output in an infant is equal to 50 per cent of its ECF, compared with 20 per cent of the ECF in an adult. The infant's kidney has a poor response to ADH. With no water intake an infant dies in 4–5 days, while a normal adult deprived of water dies in about 10 days in a temperate climate.

Some Specific Paediatric Problems

These include:

a   No protection against being given high solute diets. An infant cannot specifically complain of thirst.

b   Susceptibility to gastroenteritis, with consequent loss of fluid and electrolytes.

c   Ammonium production is low in the infant, and the development of metabolic acidosis is easier. Both the premature infant and the low birth-weight infant are born on the verge of metabolic acidosis. The body buffering capacity is lower in newborn infants.

d   The infant's food intake, containing about 750 ml of fluid, produces a further 300–350 ml, making over a litre of fluid daily. The food intake is only slightly in surplus to requirements, as growth is very rapid. The infant's basal metabolic rate is higher when compared with a normal adult.

e   The respiratory defence of plasma hydrogen ion is not as prompt as in adults, and premature infants have a slower response than normal term infants.

f   Specific conditions with loss of water and/or electrolytes:
    i   Pyloric stenosis—repeated vomiting.
    ii   Renal tubular acidosis.
    iii   Nephrogenic diabetes insipidus. [R]
    iv   Cystic fibrosis of the pancreas.
    v   Congenital potassium losers. [R]
    vi   Congenital chloride losers. [R]
    vii   Congenital absence of thirst. [R].

Clinical Signs and Symptoms

A baby is easy to weigh, and weight change can be rapidly noted. A thirsty baby will drink water, but nausea may mask thirst. The character of respiration and its rate can easily be noted. Similarly presence or absence of tears and salivation are easily seen. Beware of the 'good baby', which may in fact be apathetic, and weak.

PARATHYROID HORMONE

Parathyroid hormone is released from the parathyroid glands in response to a fall below normal of plasma ionized calcium concentration (and ? following a fall below normal of plasma inorganic phosphate) in three forms:

a Intact molecule—biologically active; $T_{\frac{1}{2}} = 20$ min.

b N-terminal fragment—biologically active; $T_{\frac{1}{2}} = 5$ min.

c C-terminal fragment—two-thirds of the intact molecule; biologically inactive; biological $T_{\frac{1}{2}} = 30$ min; estimation of the C-terminal fragment reflects the level of PTH release.

Parathyroid Hormone Activity

Stimulates osteoclast activity and increases recruitment of osteoclasts, releasing calcium and phosphate from bone into the plasma. This increase in osteoclast activity is followed by an increase in the number of osteoblasts within a few weeks. The rise in plasma calcium occurs within 15 min of PTH release or injection. PTH binds to and activates adenylate receptors in bone, and during continuous PTH infusion urine hydroxyproline excretion rises two-fold after 8 h, falling to pre-infusion levels 8 h after cessation of infusion. PTH is less able to increase bone turnover if plasma $1,25\text{-}(OH)_2D_3$ is low.

Increases renal tubular reabsorption of inorganic phosphate, sodium, bicarbonate, potassium and amino acids.

Associated with vitamin D action $(1,25\text{-}(OH)_2D_3)$ PTH increases absorption of calcium, magnesium and phosphate from the gastrointestinal tract.

PHOSPHATE

Dietary Intake

Phosphate-rich foods include eggs and milk. Of the 29–45 mmol (900–1400 mg) intake per day, 20–40 per cent is excreted in the faeces and 60–80 per cent is absorbed, and excreted in the urine. During a period of fasting, up to 4·5 mmol plasma inorganic phosphate (Pi), derived from bone, are excreted daily in the urine. After 1–2 days of fasting this urine loss drops to 1–1·8 mmol per day.

Absorption

Most of the dietary phosphate is absorbed in the jejunum, with some absorption taking place in the stomach and the rest of the small intestine. Absorption is linked to the absorption of sodium (mol for mol), and $H_2PO_4^-$ is absorbed preferentially to HPO_4^{2-} (i.e. absorption of phosphate is greater at a low pH). Parathyroid hormone and vitamin D both enhance absorption of phosphate from the jejunum. Active calcium absorption requires the presence of phosphate ions.

Plasma inorganic phosphate concentration increases after phosphate-rich foods, and a peak plasma level is reached by 1 h, with peak increment in stable phosphate by $1\frac{1}{2}$ h. After carbohydrate foods, the plasma inorganic phosphate falls, and after oral glucose (e.g. glucose tolerance test) plasma inorganic phosphate falls within 1–2 h by 0·05–0·15 mmol/l.

Functions

Phosphate is the major intracellular anion, involved in the integrity of cell water. It is a vital constituent of bone, ATP, creatine phosphate (i.e. energy storage) and red cell 2,3-DPG (oxygen carriage and release by haemoglobin).

Phosphate is the major anion buffer in the urine, as urinary titratable acid, i.e. $Na_2HPO_4 : NaH_2PO_4$.

Body Distribution

Total adult body phosphate = 19 400 mmol (600 g), predominantly in bone, muscle and other body cells. The muscle cells contain 55 mmol phosphate/kg water.

Much of the intracellular phosphate is sequestered in mitochondria and organelles as amorphous insoluble tricalcium phosphate, with release of hydrogen ions to the cytosol. An exchangeable bone phosphate pool exists, of about 100 mmol in the adult, with a slower rate of exchange than that of the ECF pool. (IC phosphate : EC phosphate = 100 : 1.)

Inorganic phosphate enters the organic phase at three points:

a. Glyceraldehyde-3-P + Pi → 1,3-diphosphoglycerate + ADP→ATP + 3-phosphoglycerate.

b. ADP + Pi→ATP.

c. During glycogenolysis with the formation of glucose-1-phosphate.

$$G\text{-}1\text{-}P \longrightarrow G\text{-}6\text{-}P$$

ECF phosphate = 19 mmol (590 mg).

Plasma Inorganic Phosphate (Pi) = 0·87–1·4 mmol/l in adults.
                                    = 1·6–2·0 mmol/l in children.

a Twelve per cent is protein-bound.

b Eighty-eight per cent is ultrafiltrable:
   i Sixty per cent is ionized.
   ii Forty per cent is complexed.

During normal adolescence, the normal plasma Pi is proportional to plasma alkaline phosphatase activity.

Plasma phospholipid = 2–6 mmol/l.

Plasma organic ester phosphate = 0·1 mmol/l.

Plasma pyrophosphate concentration is very low = 3μmol/l.

Plasma Orthophosphate Ionization in ECF

$$H_3PO_4 \rightleftharpoons H^+ + H_2PO_4^- \rightleftharpoons H^+ + HPO_4^{2-} \underset{*}{\rightleftharpoons} H^+ + PO_4^{3-}.$$

[* Negligible amounts at pH 7·4 (i.e. normal plasma pH)]
$HPO_4^{2-} : H_2PO_4^- = 4 : 1$, i.e. the apparent valence is an average of 1·8, but the valence fluctuates within the normal plasma pH range. Therefore plasma inorganic phosphate concentrations are better expressed as mmol/l (or mg/dl) rather than mEq/l.

The plasma inorganic phosphate fluctuates during the day, depending on diet etc. and therefore samples for phosphate estimation should be taken from fasting subjects.

There is a rapidly exchangeable phosphate pool of 0·6 mmol/kg body weight, with a turnover 10 times daily. This pool is twice the size of the total ECF inorganic phosphate (see points of entry of inorganic phosphate into organic phase).

Renal Excretion

Of the filtered phosphate 35–40 per cent is reabsorbed in the first 10–20 per cent of the proximal renal tubule. In the remainder of the proximal tubule, phosphate reabsorption is linked with sodium and water reabsorption, so that at the end of the proximal tubule 25 per cent of the filtered phosphate remains in the tubular lumen. In the normal subject 96 per cent of the plasma inorganic phosphate is filtered by the glomeruli. There is very little phosphate reabsorption in the loop of Henle. A further 10–25 per cent of the filtered phosphate is reabsorbed in the distal tubule by mechanisms not linked to sodium reabsorption. Five per cent of the glomerular filtrate is excreted in the urine. When the glomerular filtration rate falls below 25 ml/min, phosphate retention occurs (as in renal damage).

Hyperglycaemia decreases the tubular reabsorption of phosphate. During the buffering of hydrogen ions, each hydrogen ion entering the renal tubular lumen to be buffered by phosphate represents one bicarbonate ion released back into the circulation. $H_2PO_4^-$ moves across cell membranes by passive diffusion, but cell membranes are much less permeable to HPO_4^{2-}. The normal plasma phosphate concentration is close to the mean renal threshold for phosphate.

Renal pyrophosphate inhibits renal crystallization.

Increased Renal Phosphate Excretion

1 Acute increase in effective arterial volume.
2 Increased ECF.
3 Hyperphosphataemia.
4 Diuretics
    a Metazolamide.
    b Thiazides.
    c Frusemide.
5 Metabolic acidosis—hypercalciuria with increased phosphate clearance.
6 Potassium depletion.
7 Calcitonin action
    a Increased renal excretion of phosphate with magnesium and calcium.
    b Increased absorption of phosphate from the gut.

Reduced Phosphate Excretion

1 Reduced effective arterial volume.
2 Vitamin D action
    a Increased absorption of phosphate from the gastrointestinal tract.
    b Increased renal absorption of phosphate from the glomerular filtrate.
3 Human growth hormone administration.
4 Hypophosphataemia—with normal kidney function, there is no phosphate in the urine when the plasma inorganic phosphate level falls below 0·7 mmol/l.
5 Reduced phosphate in the diet.
    a Reduced milk, eggs and dairy products in the diet.
    b Increased intake of phosphate binder, e.g. MgO_2.

During growth the neonate retains 2·5 mmol phosphate per day (intake − output) for the first 20 years of life. After 45 years of age 1 mmol phosphate is lost on balance daily, because of involutional bone loss.

Hyperphosphataemia

Signs and Symptoms

There is enhancement of any signs and symptoms of hypocalcaemia, and there is an increased tendency to extraskeletal calcification. Production of $1,25\text{-}(OH)_2D_3$ is reduced and bone resorption is also reduced.

Causes

1. *General*

    a Increased phosphate intake ⎫
    b Increased release of intracellular ⎬ singly or in combination.
      phosphate into the ECF
    c Reduced excretion of phosphate ⎭

2. *Specific*

    a Hypoparathyroidism. Reduced renal phosphate excretion.
    b Pseudohypoparathyroidism. Reduced renal phosphate excretion.
    c Hyperthyroidism.
    d Acromegaly.
    e Decreased GFR
      i Acute renal failure.
      ii Chronic renal failure.
    When the GFR falls below 20–30 ml/min. secondary hyperparathyroidism associated with renal acidosis depresses renal phosphate excretion. With the metabolic acidosis, there is also increased release of phosphate from bone. With a further fall in the GFR the renal phosphate excretion is further reduced.
    f Increased intake of phosphate plus poor renal excretion of phosphate (cow's milk rich in phosphate given to infants).
    g Hypervitaminosis D—increased intestinal absorption of phosphate.
    h Metabolic acidosis, including lactic acidosis and diabetic keto-acidosis.
    i Respiratory acidosis.
    j Tissue ischaemia.
    k Oral or intravenous phosphate.
    l Cytotoxic therapy releasing intracellular phosphate.
    m Haemolysis—releasing phosphate from red cells.
    n Transfusion of stored blood—release of phosphate from aged cells.
    o Rhabdomyolysis—release of phosphate from muscle cells.

Treatment

1 Treatment of any acute or chronic renal failure, if possible.
2 Emergency
 a Intravenous calcium salts.
 b Intravenous glucose plus insulin—a temporary small fall in plasma inorganic phosphate follows entry of some inorganic phosphate into cells.

  c   Dialysis.

Treatment with diuretics with or without probenecid is mostly ineffective.

Hypophosphataemia
Signs and Symptoms

Symptoms do not arise until the plasma inorganic phosphate falls below 0·15 mmol/l. When plasma inorganic phosphate is less than 0·3 mmol/l it is not possible to predict the size of the body phosphate deficit. The patient suffers from malaise, lack of energy, anorexia. Central nervous system involvement includes dysarthria, hyperreflexia, paraesthesiae, tremor, ataxia, confusion and incoordination. Muscle pains, tenderness and weakness develop, which may progress to paralysis with rhabdomyolysis. Bone pains with pseudofractures visible on X-ray are related to the development of osteomalacia. There may be cardiac failure.

Erythrocyte survival is reduced, with development of spherocytosis and inability to deform (i.e. rigidity), and increased oxygen affinity with poor oxygen release to the tissues, resulting from low red cell 2,3-DPG.

Plasma creatine phosphokinase (CPK) activity increases with increasing muscle damage.

Leucocyte function is impaired with reduction in resistance to infection. Platelet function is also impaired.

Causes

1. *General*
   a   Reduced phosphate intake
   b   Increased excretion of phosphate
   c   Increased uptake of phosphate by cells
   } singly or in combination.

2. *Specific*
   a   *Decreased intestinal absorption*
      i   Low dietary phosphate.
      ii   Phosphate binders in intestinal tract, e.g. phosphate-binding antacids.
      iii   Vitamin D deficiency.
      iv   Alcoholics—poor dietary intake of phosphate-rich foods, plus increased loss of phosphate in the urine, especially during alcohol withdrawal.
   b   *Increased loss of phosphate in urine*
      i   Acute ineffective arterial volume.
      ii   Increase in ECF volume.

iii Diuretics, especially thiazides
iv Probenecid.
v   Potassium depletion—loss of potassium, magnesium, nitrogen and phosphate from cells.
vi During recovery from hypothermia.
vii During recovery phase during the treatment of diabetic ketoacidosis.
A minimum of 50 mmol of phosphate supplements are needed in the first 24 hours.
viii Hypercalcaemia, e.g. primary hyperparathyroidism.
ix Idiopathic hypercalciuria.
x   Glucagon administration.
xi Cushing's syndrome.
xii Hormone action
   α Oestrogen.
   β Androgen.
   γ Anabolic steroids.
   δ Iatrogenic glucocorticoid excess.
   ε Parathyroid hormone (decreasing renal tubular phosphate reabsorption).
xiii Severe Reye's syndrome.
xiv Renal tubule defects
   α Phosphate ± glucose loss
     a Familial hypocalcaemia.
     b Non-familial hypocalcaemia.
   β Multiple loss (Fanconi syndrome including renal tubular acidosis, Type 2)
     a Primary.
     b Secondary
       1 Genetic, e.g. cystinosis.
       2 Acquired, e.g. heavy metal poisoning.
   γ Renal hypophosphataemic metabolic bone disease
     a Sporadic
       1 Childhood onset.
       2 Adult onset.
     b Genetic
       1 X-linked dominant type.
         a Childhood onset.
         b Adult onset.
       2 Autosomal recessive type.
       3 Autosomal dominant type.
     c Acquired
       1 Tumours of bone and soft tissue.
       2 Fibrous dysplasia of bone.
       3 Epidermal naevus.

c Shift of Phosphate into Cells

   i   Recovery phase after burns.

   ii Bone repair.

  iii Hyperventilation

The reduced P_{CO_2} leads to increased intracellular pH with increased glycolysis and entry of inorganic phosphate into cells, to form phosphorylated carbohydrate compounds. After voluntary hyperventilation inorganic phosphate falls by 0·2 mmol/l returning to normal within 5 hours. Glycogen deposition in the liver is accompanied by flux of phosphate and potassium into cells.

   iv Heat stroke—plasma inorganic phosphate falls by up to 0·3 mmol/l.

   v Respiratory alkalosis (see hyperventilation).

   vi Metabolic acidosis.

  vii Salicylate poisoning.

 viii Acute gout.

   ix Gram-negative septicaemia.

   x Insulin and/or glucose administration.

   xi Androgens—incorporation of phosphate into cells.

  xii Hyperalimentation with dehydration, refeeding with protein and anabolic steroids without adequate phosphate replacement.

Treatment

1. Give enough phosphate to correct the deficit without causing side-effects, at the rate of 0·15–0·33 mmol/kg body weight intravenously over a 6-h period, checking blood levels of phosphate, calcium and potassium between each treatment. Or give 9 mmol monobasic potassium phosphate in half-strength saline by continuous infusion over 12-h, checking plasma inorganic phosphate, calcium and potassium, before repeating, if necessary. Calcium supplements may also be required.

2. At the same time, stop phosphate-binding antacid therapy; treat primary hyperparathyroidism; treat vitamin D deficiency; treat primary defects in renal tubular phosphate reabsorption with foods rich in phosphate plus oral phosphate supplements. The diagnosis of phosphate depletion is supported by the clinical improvement following phosphate replacement. Stop phosphate replacement when the plasma inorganic phosphate exceeds 0·32 mmol/l.

Loss of Intracellular Phosphate

1 Starvation.

2 Trauma and/or surgical operation.

3 Infection.

4 Potassium depletion.
5 Diabetic ketoacidosis.
6 Alcoholic ketoacidosis.
7 Hyperparathyroidism.
8 Hyperthyroidism.

POTASSIUM

Dietary Content

Anchovy paste 50 mmol/100 g
Potato crisps 33–34 mmol/100 g
Dried beans 30 mmol/100 g
Potato chips 23 mmol/100 g
Semi-dried dates 20 mmol/100 g
Peanut butter 20 mmol/100 g
Ham (less excess fat)
16 mmol/100 g

Dried prunes, peaches,
apricots 10–25 mmol/100 g
Walnuts 10 mmol/100 g
Cooked meat 8 mmol/100 g
Oranges, bananas
8 mmol/100 g

Absorption

Dietary content average = 80 mmol/day (70–100 mmol/day).
72 mmol excreted in urine.
8 mmol excreted in faeces.
Most of the ingested potassium is absorbed from the gastrointestinal tract, mainly in the small intestine.

Secretion

In the salivary glands, the initial secretion (isotonic with plasma) has a high potassium content, which is exchanged with sodium from the blood. Potassium bicarbonate is reabsorbed faster than sodium is exchanged, and the salivary secretion becomes hypotonic. Its pH is 5·5–6·0, and at peak flow the pH rises to 7·8. The secreted potassium is reabsorbed in the small intestine.

Saliva 500–1500 ml/day	Potassium up to 20 mmol/l
Gastric juice 2000–3000 ml/day	Potassium up to 10 mmol/l
Pancreatic juice	
300–1500 ml/day	Potassium up to 5 mmol/l
Bile 250–1100 ml/day	Potassium up to 5 mmol/l
Intestinal secretion approx.	Potassium up to 10 mmol/l
3000 ml/day	
Colonic fluid small volume	Potassium up to 70 mmol/l (ion concentration in faecal water after sodium re-absorption and potassium exchange).

Function

Potassium is the main intracellular ion.

Muscle Contraction

The end plate potential is associated with increased permeability to both sodium and potassium ions. The terminal part of the nerve fibre releases acetylcholine, which acts on muscle membrane. The muscle membrane is depolarized and generates an action potential in the muscle fibre. Calcium ions which enter the muscle cell are essential. Potassium ions are extruded when the muscle contracts.

Nervous Conduction

The resting cell is relatively permeable to potassium and chloride, but impermeable to sodium ions. In the active state the cell becomes temporarily more permeable to sodium than to the other ions. With entry of sodium into the cells down the sodium gradient, the membrane potential changes, with depolarization of the membrane. Returning to the resting state, sodium permeability is reduced, with a rise again in potassium permeability, and sodium is actively pumped out of the cell.

Resting muscle cell membrane proportional to

log (ICF potassium concentration/ECF potassium concentration)

The normal electric charge across the cell membrane = 90 mV with the negative charge inside the cell.

Cell membranes are almost completely impermeable to chloride ion. The potassium equilibrium potential is more negative than the resting potential across the semipermeable membrane of the cell wall. To hold potassium inside fibres by electrical forces alone, requires the resting potential = -90 mV.

In the axon at rest the cell membrane is 50 times more permeable to potassium than to sodium. The resting membrane potential depends on a sodium/potassium pump which, by setting up concentration differences, makes the establishment of a potential difference across the cell membrane possible. The precise value of the potential difference is determined by the relative permeability of the cell membrane to sodium and potassium ions.

Body Distribution (in a 70-kg man)
Intracellular Fluid

98 per cent of total body potassium—two-thirds bound, 8–15 per cent exchangeable.

Muscle 2730 (2100–3000) mmol.

Skin ⎫
Bone ⎬ 600 mmol.
Nerves ⎬
Brain ⎭
Red blood cells 200–250 mmol.
Liver 135–200 mmol.
Other 500–700 mmol.

Plasma

3·4–5·6 mmol/l (poor indicator of presence/absence or severity of potassium depletion).
    3·0–6·0 mmol/l = 'no symptoms'.
    2·5–7·0 mmol/l = 'safe range'.
Plasma pH falls by 0·1 for each rise in plasma potassium of 1 mmol/l. The distribution of potassium between ICF and ECF is affected by the acid–base balance state.

Interstitial Fluid

Potassium concentration = 4 mmol/l (in equilibrium with plasma).

Cerebrospinal Fluid

Potassium concentration = 2·0–3·0 mmol/l (potential difference between CSF and blood = +5 mV).

Extracellular Fluid

The ECF contains 56 (48–65) mmol (1·5—2 per cent of total body potassium).

Body Potassium

31–57 mmol/kg body weight = approx. 3200–3800 mmol.
    Males 45 ± 4 mmol/kg.
    Females 37 ± 3 mmol/kg.
    Potassium enters cells in the anabolic state at the rate of 2·7 mmol K per g N. 1 g N = 6·25 g protein. The formation of 1 g glycogen requires the entry of 0·33 mmol K into the cell.

Variation in Intake of Potassium

1. Reduction of Daily Potassium Intake to 'Nil'

The urinary output of potassium continues at approximately 40 mmol/day for a few days, the degree of potassium conservation depending on the body sodium content, and acid–base balance. Eventually a steady urine potassium excretion rate of 10–20 mmol/day is reached.

2. Oral Potassium Salts

Oral potassium salts are rapidly absorbed, followed by a rapid kaliuretic response, the urine excretion being greater following a large oral potassium load. Potassium is lost in the urine after oral potassium supplements, as aldosterone is released in response to the rise in plasma potassium, and the body exchangeable potassium is unaffected.

Renal Treatment of Potassium

Potassium in the glomerular filtrate is totally reabsorbed in the proximal tubule: luminal concentration = 5 mmol/l; tubular cell concentration = 140 mmol/l.

Potassium diffuses back into the lumen in the descending loop of Henle. The luminal concentration at the tip of the loop of Henle = 20–26 mmol/l.

In the ascending loop, in the thin segment potassium diffuses into the lumen, while in the thick segment reabsorption of potassium from the lumen is associated with the active reabsorption of chloride.

In the early distal tubule the luminal fluid potassium concentration = 1 mmol/l. In the distal tubule passive diffusion of potassium into the lumen occurs in exchange for active sodium reabsorption. The distal tubule luminal fluid is electronegative relative to the tubular cells, with active secretion of potassium into the lumen and active reabsorption of potassium from the luminal fluid both possible.

An increase in plasma potassium slows down hydrogen ion secretion and bicarbonate reabsorption, the plasma bicarbonate falls as the plasma pH falls. With a fall in plasma potassium, there is increased hydrogen ion secretion and increased bicarbonate reabsorption, leading to hypokalaemic alkalosis and a rise in plasma pH. Aldosterone acts on the distal tubule, increasing potassium loss. The final result is that 85 per cent of the potassium in the glomerular filtrate is reabsorbed, and up to 120 mmol of potassium are excreted in the urine each day, when a normal diet is eaten.

Effects of Changes in Plasma Hydrogen Ion Concentration
1. Acidosis

Potassium leaves cells in exchange for hydrogen ions.

2. Alkalosis

a Respiratory alkalosis—renal potassium excretion normal.

b Metabolic alkalosis—renal potassium excretion increased.

Hypokalaemia

1. Signs and Symptoms

a. General

The patient may feel nauseated and vomit. Breathlessness occurs with shallow respirations. Ileus develops. The patient is easily tired.

b. Muscle

There is muscle weakness when plasma potassium falls below 2·5 mmol/l. Abdominal distension develops with paralytic ileus, due to weakness of the plain muscle in the intestinal tract. The muscles are flabby, and reflexes become diminished and may be absent. The pulse is weak, heart sounds are faint, blood pressure falls, and cardiac failure is associated with cardiomegaly and hypotension. There is impairment of the carotid sinus reflex and vascular response to catecholamines is reduced. Cardiac arrhythmias appear. Falling intracellular potassium in muscles causes tetany, and muscle cramps occur. Finally, death occurs in ventricular diastole.

The heart muscle is abnormally sensitive to digitalis, and the ECG shows low voltage, with prolonged Q–T interval, depressed RS–T segment, T waves inverted, widened and flattened. There may be merging of T and U waves, and the U waves become more prominent and also become biphasic.

c. Kidney

When potassium depletion exceeds 200 mmol, the kidney is unable to concentrate urine normally. When the depletion exceeds 400–600 mmol, there is difficulty in increasing urine osmolality above plasma osmolality. Nocturia develops, with polyuria resistant to vasopressin (ADH).

d. Central Nervous System

Signs and symptoms include depression, drowsiness, lethargy, apathy, and irritability. With greater depletion, there may be delirium, hallucinations, fits, confusion, and finally coma.

e. Plasma Potassium Concentration

The plasma potassium concentration may fall by 1 mmol/l when the body potassium depletion reaches 100–200 mmol. When the potassium deficit reaches 200–400 mmol, the plasma potassium may fall by a further 1 mmol/l, but plasma potassium concentrations are not reliable guides to the state of potassium deficiency.

f. Metabolic Consequences of hypokalaemia

Sodium and hydrogen ions enter the cells in potassium depletion, as intracellular potassium diffuses into the ECF. Little reduction in intracellular potassium occurs until the plasma potassium concentration falls below 3 mmol/l. Even though the daily potassium intake may be greatly reduced, inevitable continued cellular catabolism results in an obligatory excretion of approximately 15 mmol of potassium per day in the urine.

Renal conservation takes up to 2–3 weeks to develop completely when the potassium intake has been drastically reduced. The kidney produces prostaglandins which antagonize the action of ADH, and which cause an ADH-resistant polyuria. Indomethacin, which inhibits prostaglandin synthesis, restores renal concentrating ability.

Increased ammonia synthesis in renal tubules occurs, with exchange in the distal renal tubule of hydrogen ions (which combine with ammonia to form ammonium) for potassium ions which are reabsorbed. This increased synthesis of ammonia may cause coma in severe liver disease. The persistent loss of hydrogen ions combined with ammonia spares potassium, but leads to alkalosis. Potassium is essential for insulin secretion, so that hypokalaemia results in reduced insulin secretion. Potassium is also essential for the release of aldosterone, and in consequence in hypokalaemia, the excretion of sodium and chloride in the urine is increased. Potassium depletion eventually increases any coincident hyponatraemia.

Loss of sodium from the body can be very rapid, as it is the major cation in the ECF, whereas potassium loss tends to be slower.

As the cell membrane potential rises in skeletal, plain and cardiac muscle, in potassium deficiency, there is hyperpolarization. The transmembrane potential differences may rise so high that initiation of an action potential is difficult, leading to paralysis, and eventually death in ventricular diastole.

2. *Causes*

    a.   Shift of Potassium from ECF into ICF

        Acute alkalosis.

        Glucose ingestion with or without insulin injection.

Insulin therapy, e.g. in the treatment of diabetes mellitus ketoacidosis.

Vigorous hyperalimentation—induction of anabolic state.

Hyperthyroid periodic paralysis, especially after large carbohydrate meal, when potassium and glucose enter the cells.

Human growth hormone ⎫
Catecholamine action ⎬ potassium enters the cells.
Androgen therapy ⎭

Familial hypokalaemic periodic paralysis during attacks.

b. True Potassium Deficiency with Reduced Plasma Potassium Levels

(The total body potassium falls in old age, due to progressive loss of muscle mass.)

Low potassium intake in diet.

Severe congestive cardiac failure—the total body potassium falls, increasing with its severity, largely accounted for by loss of muscle mass.

Gastrointestinal loss

Gastric juice loss—pyloric stenosis with vomiting; gastric aspiration.

Intestinal fluid loss—ileostomy (recent); aspiration; pancreatic watery diarrhoea (more than 200 mmol may be lost per day); pancreatic fistula.

Diarrhoea (maximum loss = 100–200 mmol/day).

Laxative abuse.

Villous adenoma.

Ileal bladder—chloride and sodium reabsorbed with potassium loss in: ureterosigmoidostomy; uretero-ileostomy.

Renal loss (when plasma $K^+ < 3$–4 mmol/l with urine $K^+ > 50$ mmol/day = renal potassium loss)

i Mineralocorticoid action

Primary and secondary hyperaldosteronism—increased urine potassium excretion in exchange for sodium and hydrogen ions. Potentiates diuretic action.

Primary adrenal hyperplasia—deoxycorticoid increased; corticosterone increased.

Administered mineralocorticoid.

Cushing's syndrome and other causes of increased ACTH action—weakness due to low plasma potassium plus anti-anabolic action of steroids on muscle.

Carbenoxolone treatment of peptic ulcer.

Liquorice administration.

ii Increased sodium delivery to the distal renal tubules and collecting ducts

Diuretics—used for induction of diuresis; used in the treatment of hypertension. A few patients treated with thiazide diuretics develop plasma potassium levels of less than 3 mmol/l. When the plasma potassium is 3·5 mmol/l, this is associated with a fall in total body potassium of approximately 200 mmol). Perhaps 15–20 per cent of patients with essential hypertension treated with thiazide diuretics develop hypokalaemia to such a degree that they require potassium supplements (? abnormal sodium/potassium flux across cell membranes). There is no gain in efficiency of treatment of hypertension if daily bendrofluazide is increased above 5 mg, or chlorthalidone above 25 mg.

Metabolic acidosis—potassium ions leave cells in exchange for hydrogen ions.

Bartter's syndrome [R]—severe hypokalaemic alkalosis without hypertension, with raised plasma renin and aldosterone, and inadequate response of arterioles to the action of angiotensin II (i.e. no hypertension). The reduced plasma volume causes a persisent hyperreninaemia. There is partial response to treatment with indomethacin.

iii Delivery of poorly absorbable anions to the distal renal nephron

Metabolic alkalosis.

Respiratory acidosis—plasma potassium falls rapidly during the treatment of acute respiratory acidosis.

Bicarbonate administration (e.g. after cardiac arrest).

Acetazolamide diuretic therapy.

Diabetic ketoacidosis.

Large doses of penicillin, carbenicillin (large molecule anions).

In alkalosis renal reabsorption of sodium and bicarbonate in exchange for hydrogen ions does not occur. Potassium is lost in place of sodium, leading to potassium deficit and 'paroxysmal aciduria', when hydrogen ions are excreted in exchange for potassium ions, to conserve potassium. Low plasma potassium levels favour alkalosis, and also favour tissue binding of digitalis glycosides.

Potassium-wasting nephritis [R]. Secondary hyper-aldosteronism results in potassium loss.

Renal tubular acidosis
Distal tubular acidosis—hypokalaemia common.
Proximal tubular acidosis—hypokalaemia occurs occasionally in the early stages.
Hypophosphataemia.
Chronic interstitial nephritis

iv Other causes
Magnesium deficiency.
Acute myelomonocytic leukaemia (high potassium load from leukaemic cell breakdown).
Excessive loss of potassium in skin sweat.
Pseudoaldosteronism (Liddle's syndrome).

3. Treatment

a Intravenous infusion of potassium salt at the rate of 10 mmol/h, keeping the concentration of potassium in the infused fluid below 40 mmol/l
 i Potassium chloride is used in the treatment of metabolic alkalosis with potassium depletion.
 ii Potassium citrate is used for the treatment of renal tubular acidosis with potassium depletion. Up to 240 mmol of potassium can be given intravenously each day, and at least 24 mmol of potassium should be given each day.

b Potassium loss in the urine should be reduced to 0–80 mmol/day
 i Reduce the dose of diuretic if possible, and consider the use of potassium-sparing diuretics.
 ii Potassium secretion in the distal tubule depends on the sodium load delivered to the distal tubule. Therefore salty foods should be avoided, and salt should not be added at meals.

c Oral potassium supplements. Each two 'slow-K' tablets per day only raise the plasma potassium concentration by +0·1 mmol/l. A rise in plasma potassium following oral potassium salt results in increased glomerular filtrate potassium, which in turn stimulates formation and release of aldosterone. Aldosterone activates sodium/potassium ATPase, the potential difference across the distal renal tubule cells is increased, which results in increased sodium reabsorption and passive potassium loss into the urine. There is also increased permeability of the distal renal tubule cells to both sodium and potassium. Thus oral potassium salt supplements are probably lost in the urine. More effective potassium supplements consist of potassium-rich foods.

d Patients treated with corticosteroids, ACTH or carbenoxolone, usually require potassium supplements, if they are treated with diuretics.

Hyperkalaemia
Signs and Symptoms

The signs and symptoms are worse, the faster the plasma potassium concentration rises. The potassium concentration in the plasma in relation to the plasma concentrations of calcium, sodium and magnesium, determine the degree of change in the ECG.

The patient may complain of weakness, cramps, muscle pain and colic. There may be diarrhoea, with nausea, irritability and dizziness.

Muscle paralysis develops, moving centripetally, and eventually causing respiratory failure. As the plasma potassium concentration rises, muscle cells become partly depolarized, and hence less excitable, which may lead to cardiac muscle atony. ECG changes may appear when the plasma potassium level exceeds 5·5 mmol/l. With increasing hyperkalaemia the following changes occur:

a High peaked T-waves with narrow bases, especially in the precordial leads.
b P–R and QRS intervals are increased, with atrioventricular and interventricular block.
c P waves are lost.
d S–T segment is raised.
e Arrhythmia.
f Ventricular fibrillation.
g Death in systole.

Causes
a. Pseudohyperkalaemia
  i Thrombocytosis.
  ii Leucocytosis.
  iii In vitro leakage of potassium from red cells.
     (i), (ii) and (iii) Intracellular potassium tends to leak out of white cells, platelets and red cells, if blood clots and the resulting serum is used for potassium estimation, and if plasma or serum is not separated from the red cells soon after collection of the sample.

b. True Hyperkalaemia
  i *Shift of potassium from ICF to ECF*
     α Acidosis.

β   Intravascular haemolysis.
γ   Crush injury. Muscle is very rich in potassium.
δ   Succinylcholine used during anaesthesia on patients with
    paralysed muscle.
ε   Cationic amino acid therapy
    a   Including lysine, arginine, epsilon-aminocaproic acid.
    b   Hyperalimentation.
ζ   Familial hyperkalaemia periodic paralysis [R], [AD], during
    attacks of paralysis. These attacks are precipitated by
    muscle exercise and a carbohydrate-rich diet.
η   Severe dehydration.

ii *Decreased excretion of potassium*
    α   Diabetes mellitus—reduced aldosterone release and ab-
        sence of aldosterone feedback mechanism.
    β   Aldosterone deficiency
        a   Addison's disease.
        b   Selective aldosterone deficiency.
        c   Renal tubules non-responsive to aldosterone
              i   Spironolactone therapy.
              ii   Pseudoaldosteronism (Liddle's syndrome [R]).
              iii Hyporeninaemia.
    γ   Type IV renal tubular acidosis. A condition with low plasma
        renin and low plasma aldosterone.
    δ   Renal retention of potassium
        a   Potassium-sparing diuretics
              i   Amiloride.
              ii   Triamterene.
        b   Renal failure—hydrogen ions are retained and enter cells,
              displacing potassium ions into the ECF in early uraemic
              acidosis.
        c   Severe dehydration.

iii *Increased potassium intake*
    It is possible to take dangerously large doses of these salts in
    large enough volumes of fluid to avoid the normal protective
    vomiting which follows the drinking of strong salt solutions.
    Excessive intake of potassium salts is obviously more dangerous
    if there is also renal impairment. Penicillin G contains 1·7 mmol
    per million units. Hyperkalaemia may complicate
    hyperalimentation.

iv *Normal anion gap metabolic acidosis*
    The plasma potassium concentration may be normal or raised.
    α   Hyperalimentation.
    β   Post-hypocapnoea.
    γ   Dilutional acidosis.
    δ   Hypoaldosteronism.

    a Adrenal damage.
    b Failure of renal tubules to respond to aldosterone.
    c Hyporeninaemia.
    ε Intravenous arginine.
    ζ Ammonium chloride load.
    η Early uraemic acidosis.

Treatment
Emergency

1. Ten ml of 10 per cent calcium gluconate i.v. over 5 min. The calcium probably binds to the plasma cell membrane and alters the intramembrane potential. The response to hyperkalaemia is within 2 min and lasts 15–120 min.
2. Sodium bicarbonate to correct acidosis, 45 mmol as i.v. bolus, or 90 mmol in 500 ml 10 per cent dextrose in water. The response to hyperkalaemia occurs within 5 min and the effects last some hours.
3. Fifty ml of 50 per cent glucose plus 10 units of regular insulin i.v. should bring the plasma potassium concentration down by 1·5 mmol/l in 15–30 min.

    The plasma sodium, potassium, chloride and bicarbonate concentrations should be checked after treatment, along with plasma PCO_2, pH and base excess.

Emergency Treatment should be followed by
Ten per cent glucose in physiological saline.
Repeat 45 mmol sodium bicarbonate i.v. over 5 min, if acidosis still present.
Sodium polystyrene sulphonate—150 g t.d.s. orally with 20 ml
                         70 per cent sorbitol.
                 —50 g in 200 ml water as
                      retention enema every 45 min.
9-alpha-fluorocortisone 0·1–0·2 mg per day.
Potassium-losing diuretics.
If the plasma potassium concentration persists above 7 mmol/l, then peritoneal or renal dialysis is indicated.

RENIN

Renin is a proteolytic enzyme which is produced and stored in the juxtaglomerular cells surrounding the afferent arterioles supplying the corresponding glomerulus of cortical glomeruli. The juxtaglomerular cells detect the degree of change of stretch in the afferent arteriolar walls, a reflection of blood pressure, and the macula densa cells possibly monitor the sodium or osmolar concentration in the proximal and distal renal tubular fluids.

Renin has a molecular weight of 40000 daltons, and it acts on angiotensinogen to release angiotensin I (*see* synthesis of aldosterone, p. 5).

Low or high plasma renin levels do not appear to affect the clinical outcome in hypertensive patients.

1 *Reduction in mean renal arterial pressure leading to renin release*
   a Upright posture assumed and maintained ⎱
   b Haemorrhage ⎰ vasoconstriction
   c Reduction in ECF ⎱ with aldosterone
   d Cardiac output falling ⎰ release.
   e Prevention of venous return to the heart.
   f Constriction of the aorta.
   g Constriction of the renal artery.
2 *Other causes of renin release*
   a Sympathetic nerve stimulation.
   b Decreased plasma potassium.
   c Beta-catecholamines.
   d Increased salt intake.
   e Diuretics
      i Volume depletion.
      ii Salt reabsorption inhibited.
      iii Reduced salt delivery to the macula densa.
      iv Direct action of diuretics on release mechanism.
   f Ureteral obstruction.
(Haemangiopericytoma is rich in renin.)
3 *Conditions with high renin and low aldosterone*
   a Generalized adrenocortical insufficiency.
   b Primary adrenal defect, with selective aldosterone deficiency.
   c Renal tubule unresponsiveness to aldosterone, pseudo-hypoaldosteronism, Liddle's disease.
   d Potassium-sparing diuretics.
   e Adrenal ablation ⎱
   f Cushing's disease ⎰ lack of feedback.
   g Adrenocortical insufficiency (Addison's disease) ⎰ feedback.
4 *Renin release suppressed*
   a Low salt intake.
   b Potassium intake increased.
   c Action of angiotensin II (negative feedback action following renin release).
   d Action of ADH.
5 *Conditions with low plasma renin and low aldosterone*
   a Hyporeninaemic hypoaldosteronism
      i Mild renal insufficiency—diabetic nephropathy.
          —gouty nephropathy.
          —other nephropathies.

ii   In the absence of renal disease [R].
Plasma potassium concentration can be maintained at normal level if a liberal intake of salt is possible.

CONTROL OF RESPIRATION

The medullary rhythmicity centre (area) controls the automatic rate of respiration. For variations in the rate and depth of respiration a 'dual centre concept' has been put forward:

a. One centre not protected by the blood–brain barrier, and therefore readily influenced by changes in hydrogen ion concentration or bicarbonate concentration in the circulating blood.

b. Second centre protected by blood–brain barrier, and therefore only slowly affected by changes in hydrogen ion or bicarbonate ion concentrations. Carbon dioxide, which freely penetrates membranes, will be able to stimulate this centre rapidly.

It is thought that 20–40 per cent of the respiratory drive is normally controlled by peripheral chemoreceptors, and this drive is increased markedly by hypoxaemia or acidaemia, and

$$H^+ = K'.\frac{CO_2}{HCO_3{}^-}.$$

Increased Respiration during Normal Exercise

a. It is suggested that receptors are activated by movements of limbs and possibly contraction of muscles, which stimulate increased breathing during exercise (not chemosensitive), *or*

b. Exercise hyperpnoea originates from a cerebrocortical centre (to explain the sudden increase in breathing during exercise).

Dyspnoea

Stimulation of the medullary respiratory centre.
Hypersensitivity of the Hering–Breuer reflex, which brings about an earlier inhibition of the inspiratory phase of respiration, resulting in rapid shallow breathing. The problems of respiration in dyspnoea are complicated.

SODIUM
Dietary Intake
An average daily diet contains 100–200 mmol.

Absorption

Normally all ingested sodium is absorbed from the gastrointestinal tract. There is little sodium absorption from the stomach, and some 'neutral' sodium and potassium chloride is secreted into the gastric juices. The osmolality between the stomach contents and the plasma is equalized in the jejunum. There is free movement of water in both directions across the mucous membranes of both the small and large intestines, with less movement across the gastric mucosa. Absorption of sodium in the jejunum is against a small gradient. In the presence of bicarbonate there is active sodium absorption, which also depends on active absorption of glucose in the small intestine. There is a greater gradient in the ileum, with decreasing concentration of sodium in the lumen as the caecum is approached. Fifty mmol sodium are absorbed daily in the colon ionically associated with secretion of potassium, with simultaneous absorption of chloride in exchange for bicarbonate, enhanced by the action of aldosterone. Only 1–10 mmol of sodium are excreted daily in the faeces. Sodium is actively secreted in the pancreatic juice, bile and succus entericus, subsequently being completely reabsorbed lower down the small and large intestines.

Sodium Absorption reduced

   a.   Diarrhoea.
   b.   Intestinal obstruction just distal to the duct of Wirsung, resulting in pancreatic and gastric juice loss.
   c.   Action of gastrin and related gastrointestinal hormones.
   d.   Cholera toxin—active sodium bicarbonate loss in watery stools.

Functions

Sodium is the major extracellular cation. In the active state sodium permeates into the nerve cell and the muscle cell. Sodium is pumped out of cells by sodium/potassium-dependent ATPase pump in cell membranes, with energy derived from the breakdown of ATP, and sodium crosses the cell membrane linked with protein.

Sodium Ions enter Cells

   1. When the sodium pumps in cell membranes are impaired, e.g. congenital spherocytic haemolytic anaemia.
   2. In severe potassium deficiency, potassium ions are lost from cells, and probably some sodium and hydrogen ions enter the cells, although not to the degree postulated in the sick cell syndrome.
   3. When the intracellular hydrogen ion concentration falls (i.e. pH rises), sodium ions may enter cells.

Body Distribution

Total body sodium—40–60 mmol/l, i.e. 5000 mmol in a 70-kg man.
   —60–70 per cent rapidly exchangeable.
   —up to 40 per cent non-exchangeable, bound
      to bone matrix and other sites.
ICF sodium approximately
   10 mmol/l—2 per cent of total sodium (270 mmol).
ECF sodium approximately
   150 mmol/l—2100 mmol.
      —plasma sodium 11 per cent.
      —ISF sodium 30 per cent of total.

Normal plasma sodium = 135–147 mmol/l.

Normal saliva—20 mmol/l (700–1000 ml per day).
Gastric juices—varies with acid secretion.
Small intestines—140 mmol/l with 10–20 mmol/l of potassium.
Normal stool—20 mmol/l.
Cerebrospinal fluid sodium—135–143 mmol/l.

Renal Excretion

The urinary excretion of sodium normally equals the dietary intake which is totally absorbed. If the sodium intake is reduced to nil, then with normal renal function, urinary sodium output rapidly falls to nil.

The glomerular filtrate contains 140×180 mmol/day—approximately 25 200 mmol/day; 50–70 per cent of this sodium load is reabsorbed in the proximal renal tubule isosmotically with chloride and bicarbonate ions. In the ascending loop of Henle a further 25 per cent of the sodium load is passively reabsorbed with actively reabsorbed chloride ions. Finally in the distal renal tubule and collecting duct, a further 5 per cent is reabsorbed, the rate of reabsorption being controlled by the action of aldosterone.

Ninety-nine per cent of the filtered sodium is reabsorbed.

Urine Sodium Excretion

Ranges from 1–5 mmol/l to 200 mmol/l, with a daily total excretion range of from '0' to 340 mmol/day.

Alterations in the sodium concentration in the plasma entering the carotid artery affect the carotid bodies, and hence affect the rate of sodium excretion. Increase in sodium concentration in the plasma entering the liver causes increased urinary sodium excretion, this effect being abolished by vagotomy. There is marked sodium retention in the Budd–Chiari syndrome.

Increased Urinary Sodium Loss

1 Diuretics.
2 Osmotic diuresis—glucose,
           —mannitol.
3 Metabolic acidosis.
4 Relief of urinary obstruction.
5 Diuretic phase of recovery after acute renal tubular necrosis.
6 Adrenal insufficiency.
7 'Salt-losing' renal disease
   a Pyelonephritis.
   b Cystic disease of the kidney.
   c Renal tubular acidosis.

Hyponatraemia

Signs and Symptoms

Hyponatraemia may be symptomless, especially in young children and in the elderly. The severity of signs and symptoms of hyponatraemia are proportional to the degree of hyponatraemia, and also to the rate of its development. An abrupt fall in plasma sodium from 140 mmol/l to 125 mmol/l is associated with developing mental confusion, whereas a slow fall from plasma sodium of 140 mmol/l to 125 mmol/l is well tolerated. When plasma sodium falls below 120 mmol/l, stupor, coma, seizures may develop.

Sodium deficit = $0.6 \times$ body weight(kg) $\times$ (140–observed plasma sodium (mmol/l)).

Causes

a. Pure Water Excess

In normal subjects the plasma sodium only falls when the rate of intake of water approaches 36 litres per 24 h. Up to this limit, normal renal excretion of water equals the intake. Vomiting prevents excess water intake, but antiemetics (e.g. chlorpromazine) enables excessive water intake to occur without vomiting. In older subjects the maximal rate of renal excretion of water falls, and hence tolerance of water loading also falls.

b. Extrarenal Sodium Loss with Access to Water (Urinary Sodium less than 20 mmol/l)

Gastrointestinal loss
    Gastric aspiration, vomiting.
    Intestinal fistula, intestinal drainage.
    Malfunctioning ileostomy.

Severe diarrhoea.
Skin loss
Exposure to heat.
Cystic fibrosis with abnormally high sweat sodium output.
Adrenal insufficiency—high plasma ADH with inability to excrete
water load.
Burns.
Inflammatory disease of the skin.
Other sources of sodium loss
Severe haemorrhage.
Rapid removal of large volumes of serous cavity fluid, e.g. ascites.
Extensive limb trauma.

c. *Dilutional (Low EAV)*
Nephrosis.
Cirrhosis.
Congestive cardiac failure.
Oedema.
'3rd space loss'
Ileus (intestinal).
Peritonitis.
Pancreatitis.

d. *Renal Sodium Loss (Urinary Sodium greater than 20 mmol/l)*
Renal failure. When GFR < 10 ml/min, urinary sodium excretion
range = 33–133 mmol/day
Salt wasting
Relief of urinary tract obstruction.
Nephrocalcinosis.
Interstitial nephritis.
Medullary cystic disease of the kidney.
Prerenal
Diuresis.
Mineralocorticoid deficiency.
Fasting.
Bartter's syndrome [R].
Aldosterone deficiency.
With apparently normal EAV
SIADH (water excess).
Myxoedema. GFR is reduced, less sodium is filtered, renal medul-
lary blood flow falls, and the urine sodium excretion is reduced.
Hypopituitarism.
Rest 'osmostat'.
Salt loss with water repletion.

e. Hyperosmolar Hyponatraemia

After mannitol infusion before diuresis starts.
Severe hyperglycaemia.

f. Pseudohyponatraemia

Hyperlipidaemia, as in severe diabetic ketoacidosis. When untreated lipaemic plasma is run through a flame photometer the lipid portion contains no sodium and the sodium concentration is estimated from the total plasma volume rather than from the water phase. This error is demonstrated by disparity between the estimated and calculated plasma osmolality.

Hyperproteinaemia, as in severe myeloma, or macroglobulinaemia. Again, this error can be demonstrated by the disparity between the estimated and the calculated plasma osmolality.

Treatment

1 Treat the cause.
2 Reduce or discontinue salt-losing diuretics.
3 Replace mineralocorticoids, glucocorticoids, or thyroid hormone as indicated.
4 Hypervolaemia requires reduction in salt and water intake, with daily water intake less than the sum of insensible loss plus urine output.
5 In endocrine hyponatraemia restrict water intake to less than 1 litre/day.
6 In SIADH restrict water intake to less than 1 litre/day. Consider giving demeclocycline 900–1200 mg/day, with especial care in cirrhotics in whom kidney damage may occur.
   An intravenous bolus of frusemide (40 mg) may be given, and when diuresis has started, 200 ml of 5 per cent saline may be given per hour for 2–3 h. This must be very carefully supervised, as rapid changes in plasma (and ECF) sodium concentration are dangerous. Such treatment may be needed to bring the plasma sodium concentration above 120 mmol/l. Above this level water intake restriction may be all that is necessary, and is far safer.
7 Hyponatraemia with dehydration
   Intravenous isotonic saline is given slowly, the central venous pressure being kept below 16 mmHg. Gross hypoalbuminaemia is partially corrected with intravenous albumin solution, but not more than 50 g of albumin should be given during the first 24 hours of recovery.

Hypernatraemia

Signs and Symptoms

1 Lethargy progressing to coma.
2 Muscle rigidity, tremor, myoclonus, spasticity and hyperreflexia.
3 Transient generalized chorea which may progress to convulsions.
5 CSF protein concentration increased without pleocytosis.
6 Permanent brain damage has been found in infants who recover following severe hypernatraemia.

(Plasma sodium concentration exceeding 144 mmol/l is the lowest level at which there is invariably an increase in plasma vasopressin and also in urine concentration in normal adults.)

Causes

1 Absolute increase in body sodium
   Hypertonic saline infusion.
   Excess salt tablets with antiemetic.
   Hypertonic sodium bicarbonate infusion (past-cardiac arrest, or lactic acidosis).
   Excessive concentration of sodium in dialysis fluid.
2 Primary decrease in body water with normal body sodium
   Pure water loss with sodium retention
      Accute diabetes insipidus.
      Unattended comatose patient.
   Lack of access to water
      Unattended comatose patient.
      Desert ⎫
      Sea   ⎭ without available fresh water.
3 Greater loss of body water than body sodium
   Severe osmotic diuresis
      Mannitol.
      Urea.
      Glucose. ICF water is drawn from the cells into the ECF in hyperglycaemia, diluting plasma sodium.
   Severe
      Diarrhoea ⎫
      Sweating   ⎭ especially in young children.

Treatment

Restore the circulatory volume.
Aim to reduce plasma sodium with fluid replacement by *not more than* 4 mmol/l/4 h.

(The Hickey–Hare or Carter–Robins test, in which 500 ml of 3 per cent sodium chloride solution are infused intravenously to detect diabetes insipidus, is now obsolete, as the results obtained are often equivocal, and better and safer tests are available.)

THIRST

The sensation of thirst results in the drinking of water if it is available (or drinks containing water). Thirst results from a decrease in cellular hydration, following an increase in plasma osmolality. An increase in plasma osmolality of +2 per cent results in a sensation of thirst. Hypovolaemia also results in the feeling of thirst. Pleasantness of the taste of the available liquid and of the environment greatly influences the degree of thirst due to minimal cellular dehydration.

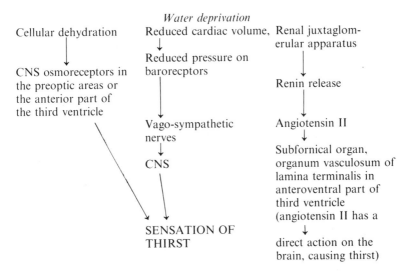

Water deprivation

Cellular dehydration → CNS osmoreceptors in the preoptic areas or the anterior part of the third ventricle

Reduced cardiac volume, Reduced pressure on barorecptors → Vago-sympathetic nerves → CNS

Renal juxtaglomerular apparatus → Renin release → Angiotensin II → Subfornical organ, organum vasculosum of lamina terminalis in anteroventral part of third ventricle (angiotensin II has a direct action on the brain, causing thirst)

SENSATION OF THIRST

Relief from Sensation of Thirst

After drinking water (fluid)
   Oropharyngeal stimulation.
   Gastric distension.
   Intestinal stimulation.
   Dilution of ECF, with fall in osmolality.

Pathological States

1   Excessive thirst.
2   Depressed thirst.

Increased Thirst

Shortage of available water.

Contracted ICF of osmoreceptors due to hyperosmolality of the ECF.

Decreased arterial pressure in the carotid artery due to reduced ECF volume or reduced cardiac output.

Decreased tension in the left atrial wall and great pulmonary veins:
Blood loss.
Prolonged quiet standing.
Positive-pressure respiration.

Pain.

Increased temperature of blood flowing through hypothalamus.

Drugs
Acetylcholine.
Morphine.
Barbiturates.
Nicotine.
Adrenergic drugs.

Stimulation of the carotid body chemoreceptors by hypoxia and/or hypercapnoea.

Stimulation of the renin–angiotensin system.

Psychosis.

Decreased Thirst

Recent drink of adequate amount of water.

Expanded ICF of neurons of supraoptic hypophyseal nuclei, secondary to hypo-osmolality of the ECF (e.g. nausea associated with hyponatraemia).

Increased arterial pressure in the carotid arteries.

Increased left atrial wall tension and increased tension in the great pulmonary veins.

Decreased temperature of blood flowing through the hypothalamus.

Drugs
Alcohol.
Phenytoin.
Narcotic antagonists.
Anticholinergics.
Atropine.

Destruction of thirst centre.

Psychosis.

TRACE ELEMENTS

1. Copper

Iron can only be transported in the ferric state. Caeruloplasmin, which is a ferroxidase, is required to oxidize ferrous storage iron to the ferric state for transport.

Severe copper deficiency can be associated with anaemia and scorbutic bone changes.

2. Zinc

Zinc is a component of many key proteins, and is released only during general protein catabolism (e.g. after surgery, trauma or severe infection). Many of the enzymes involved in nucleic acid and protein metabolism are zinc metalloproteins, e.g. thymidine kinase, and RNA and DNA polymerases.

3. Selenium

Selenium is needed for incorporation into glutathione peroxidase.

4. Chromium

Traces of chromium are required in glocuse and insulin metabolism.

5. Vanadium

Vanadate may control the response of the sodium/potassium pump in cell membranes to potassium concentration.

UREA

The normal blood ammonia level is kept very low, as free ammonia is extremely toxic (24–48 µmol/l). Amine groups derived from aminoacids, from protein, enter the Krebs urea cycle in the cytoplasm and mitochondria of the liver cells, where non-toxic urea is synthesized, with incidental release of hydrogen ions. Thus on a normal diet the urine pH is approximately 6·0.

On a normal diet about 15–20 g urea are produced per day (250–330 mmol/day).

On a carbohydrate-fat diet without protein, the daily urine urea excretion falls to 5 g (83 mmol/day), representing the continuous catabolism of body protein.

On a high-protein diet the urine excretion of urea rises to about 30 g/day (500 mmol/day). The ability to concentrate urine is reduced on a low-protein diet, and is increased on a high protein diet, the urine urea and sodium excretion rates being inversely related.

Urea diffuses passively and slowly into cells, and out again, depending on the fluxes across the cell membranes. This property has been used to reduce cerebral oedema, 30–60 g urea orally in 250 ml fluid draw water out of swollen oedematous brain cells, but it has since been found that intravenous mannitol solution is quicker and more effective.

Renal Excretion

Urea is filtered in the glomerular filtrate, and at the upper limit of water diuresis 30–40 per cent of filtered urea is reabsorbed (60–70 per cent being excreted). During antidiuresis only 15–20 per cent of the filtered urea is excreted.

If fluid intake is suddenly increased, then the urea excretion temporarily rises to very high rates, falling rapidly, the initially high urea concentration in the medulla falling. If a maintained diuresis is discontinued, urea output is temporarily very low, until the urea concentration in the medulla has risen again.

Recirculation of Urea in the Kidney

The urine entering the early distal renal tubule has a low osmolality with a low urea concentration. Water is removed progressively along the distal tubule. In antidiuresis, with urine osmolality reaching 1200 mosmol/l in the collecting ducts, and urea concentration in the medullary collecting ducts at its highest, urea diffuses freely into the interstitium to enter the sluggishly flowing blood in the vasa recta, to enter the thick ascending loop of Henle (while active chloride and passive sodium reabsorption is taking place). Again, urea diffuses out of the ascending loop into the interstitium and slowing flowing blood in the vasa recta related to the loop of Henle, eventually re-entering the tubular lumen through the cells of the pars recta of the anterior descending tubule, to recirculate down the lumen to the distal tubule once more.

The ability to concentrate urine maximally depends on the high urea and sodium chloride concentration deep in the renal medulla, and the varying permeability of the various parts of the nephron to water, urea, plus the active reabsorption or secretion of anions and cations at various sites on the nephron.

VITAMIN D

Ergosterol derived from plant foods is converted by ultraviolet light to ergocalciferol, and 7-dehydrocholesterol from animal foods is converted by ultraviolet light in the skin to cholecalciferol.

These two calciferols are converted in the liver to $25\text{-}(OH)_2D_2$ and $25\text{-}(OH)_2D_3$, respectively.

Stimulated by parathyroid hormone action, the kidney converts these latter substances to the active forms—$1,25\text{-}(OH)_2D_2$ and $1,25\text{-}(OH)_2D_3$ which have identical actions in the human body:
1. Acting with parathyroid hormone $1,25\text{-}(OH)_2D$ stimulates bone resorption with release of calcium and phosphate into the plasma. $24,25\text{-}(OH)_2D_3$ may be concerned with bone formation.
2. Stimulating absorption of calcium, magnesium, inorganic phosphate from the gastrointestinal tract. It stimulates the formation of mRNA in the intestinal mucosa with the formation of calcium-binding protein.
3. Increasing renal tubular reabsorption of calcium and inorganic phosphate, although $25\text{-}(OH)_2D$ is more effective than $1,25\text{-}(OH)_2D$ in increasing inorganic phosphate reabsorption.
4. ? Vitamin D metabolite acts on muscle. In vitamin D deficiency and osteomalacia there is often weakness of proximal muscles of the limbs.

When plasma ionized calcium concentrations are normal, the release of parathyroid hormone is stopped, and the kidney converts $25\text{-}(OH)_2D$ to the inactive form of $24,25\text{-}(OH)_2D$.

Conversion of $25\text{-}(OH)_2D$ to $1,25\text{-}(OH)_2D$ is inhibited by high concentrations of phosphate in the renal cells (e.g. in late renal failure), and is inhibited by the action of calcitonin.

Vitamin D Deficiency

1 During active growth, especially during the first two years of life, and especially during the growth rate of puberty.
   Rickets—disordered bone growth with bone distortion; hypotonia of muscles; tetany.
2 In adults after cessation of bone growth—osteomalacia.
   Hypotonia of muscles ⎫
   Bone distortion   ⎬ when hypocalcemia occurs in the absence of renal failure.
   Tetany   ⎭

Biochemical Findings—raised alkaline phosphatase, with serum calcium and phosphate normal or low.

Vitamin D Excess

Extraskeletal calcification, including calcification in kidneys.
Metabolic alkalosis with distal tubule renal acidosis (RTA Type 2).
Hypercalcaemia.

EFFECTIVE ARTERIAL VOLUME (EAV)

The blood pressure is controlled by a product of cardiac output (stroke volume × heart rate) and the peripheral vascular resistance, which in turn is affected by:

1   Intrinsic physical characteristics of vessel resistance.
2   Neuromuscular influence on vascular smooth muscle, affected by:

> Noradrenaline ⎫
> Angiotensin II ⎭ causing vasoconstriction.

> Acetylcholine ⎫
> Prostaglandins ⎬ causing vasodilatation.
> Kinins ⎭

The *effective circulating volume* is regulated by:
Vascular resistance.
Cardiac function.
Renal sodium and water excretion.

1. Reduction in Effective Circulating Volume

Reduction is followed by reduced perfusion primarily of the cortical ('salt-losing') nephrons and maintained perfusion of the juxtamedullary ('salt-retaining') nephrons. Reduced ECV results in sodium retention. This may occur after:

a   Haemorrhage.
b   Severe fluid loss.
c   Hypotension.
d   Reduced EAV with increased cardiac output occurs in conditions with a rapid arteriovenous shunt:
   i   Reduced peripheral vascular resistance.
   ii   Massive blood flow through bone in severe Paget's disease.
   iii   Increased blood flow through skin, spleen and intrapulmonary anastomoses in cirrhosis of the liver.
   iv   Dilated peripheral capillary beds in cyanotic heart disease.
   v   Arteriovenous fistula.

In these circumstances the activation of the sympathetic nervous system enables diversion of blood flow to:

a   Lungs ⎫
b   Heart ⎬ in preference to the other
c   Brain ⎭ organs in the body.
d   Muscles of respiration ⎠

There is a linear correlation between plasma osmolality and plasma ADH levels (i.e. ADH release), but the correlation slope is much steeper when the EAV is reduced—a small increase in osmolality results in a larger release of ADH.

2. Increase in Effective Circulating Volume

Increase in the EAV results in increased stretch of left atrial stretch receptors with atrial distension, followed by vagal stimulation. This results in reduced ADH release (e.g. diuresis follows an attack of paroxysmal tachycardia with increase in left atrial pressure). Similarly, the aortic arch and carotid sinuses are stimulated by stretch, resulting also in inhibition of ADH release, following activity along the parasympathetic fibres of the vagus and glossopharyngeal nerves. Increased EAV is associated with sodium retention. When there is reduced renal plasma flow with no change and no change in the GFR, there is enhanced proximal renal tubular sodium reabsorption. This occurs in:

a Congestive cardiac failure (with reduced cardiac output).
b Peripheral and splanchnic pooling of blood
   i   Cirrhosis with ascites ⎫
   ii Nephrosis   ⎬ with oedema.
   iii Congestive cardiac failure ⎭
   iv Hypoalbuminaemia
     α Nephrosis.
     β Cirrhosis.

There is a glomerulotubular balance of sodium if circulatory changes only occur slowly, so that reabsorption of sodium varies with the filtration rate. The mechanisms involved in this are still not fully understood.

WATER

Dietary Intake

In temperate climates an average 3000-calorie diet consists of:
1 450 ml of water in the food.
2 300–450 ml of water of oxidation. 10–15 ml of water are produced per 100 calories released.
3 Fluids drunk. The fluid intake is regulated by availability and by the thirst mechanism.

Absorption

Water is absorbed both from the small and large intestines, where there is free movement in both directions. There is less water transfer across the gastric mucous membrane. In the stomach and the jejunum the osmotic pressure across the mucous membrane is equalized with that of plasma.

Sodium is actively absorbed, and sodium secreted into the stomach is reabsorbed with water in the small intestine. Water absorption is enhanced by the presence of glucose, the rate of absorption of water being increased by a high sodium luminal concentration.

The maximum rate of fluid absorption can reach 20–30 litres per day, limited by the protective action of vomiting. The GFR can reach 30 ml/min, which is approximately 20–30 litres per day, with a concentration of 40 mosmol/l (sp. gr. = 1·004). It is therefore possible but difficult for a normal subject to induce water intoxication by deliberately drinking excessive volumes of fluid. As renal damage progresses in patients, water intoxication becomes a serious risk.

Total body water = approximately 55 per cent of the body weight. For obese subjects this should be reduced by 10 per cent, and increased by +10 per cent for lean subjects. Women contain 10 per cent less water than men.

There is a dynamic equilibrium:

$$ICF \rightleftharpoons ECF \quad and \quad ICF_v : ECF_v = 2 : 1$$
$$ISF \rightleftharpoons IVF$$

In a 70-kg man, e.g., the fluid distribution would be:

1   ICF = 33 per cent = 23 litres
2   ISF = 12 per cent = 8·5 litres
3   Plasma water = 4·5 per cent = 3 litres
4   Connective tissue water = 4·5 per cent = 3 litres
5   Bone water = 4·5 per cent = 3 litres
6   Transcellular water = 1·5 per cent = 1 litre

Up to 8 litres of fluid are secreted into and reabsorbed from the gastrointestinal tract each day, and 180 litres of fluid are filtered through the glomeruli, 99 per cent of this being reabsorbed. The link between these massive recyclings of water is the 3500 ml of plasma, which in turn, is in dynamic equilibrium with the ISF and the ICF.

Transcellular Fluid—secretions:

1   Saliva.
2   Gastric juices.
3   Intestinal secretions.
4   Bile.
5   Pancreatic secretions.
6   Fluid in renal tract.
7   Gonadal fluid.
8   Aqueous humour of the eye.
9   CSF.

ICF

The ICF totals about 27 litres in a 70-kg man. It contains some protein and hyaluronic acid and therefore exerts some osmotic pressure effect.

The ICF concentration of anion is 1·05 times the concentration of anion in plasma, and the ICF concentration of cation is 0·95 times the concentration of cation in plasma, because protein at a pH of 7·4 behaves as an anion.
The anion equivalence of protein = g/dl × 2·43 mmol/l.

Water elimination

1. The *osmolal clearance* is the volume of urine excreted per day which is necessary to excrete all the contained solute at an osmolality equivalent to that of plasma.
2. The *obligatory urine output* is equal to 20 per cent of the ECF in adults, but equivalent to 50 per cent of the ECF in an infant (500–800 ml and approximately 300 ml per day respectively).
3. *Free water clearance* is the difference between the total daily urine volume and the osmolal clearance, i.e. the volume of urine from which theoretically all solute has been removed during the formation of a protein-free urine of sp. gr. 1·010, or osmolality of 295 mosmol/l. The free water clearance must equal (water intake – insensible loss) to maintain normal plasma tonicity. When there is positive free water excretion, the final urine must be more dilute than the original plasma filtrate.
4. *Water loss* includes:
   a   Urine. Range of normal output: 600 ml–30 litres per day.
   b   Insensible perspiration 350–700 ml per day
   Skin water loss is especially high in pre-term babies of less than 30 weeks gestation during the first few days, as their skin is poorly keratinized. Babies weighing less than 1 kg lose both body heat and water dangerously during the first 24 hours. Methods used to avoid this include.
   i   Increased ambient humidity—there is a greater risk of infection, and visibility is poor in incubators.
   ii   Transparent plastic covering or thermal blanket.
   iii   Paraffin mixture (80 per cent soft, 20 per cent hard paraffin) applied to the skin reduces water loss by 40–60 per cent for over 6 hours after application. Unfortunately some babies develop rashes.
   c   Sensible perspiration up to 4 litres per day containing up to 30–90 mmol sodium chloride per day. During heavy work in heat, 2 litres of sweat can be lost per hour. With acclimatization to heat and humidity, sodium chloride loss falls to 2–5 mmol/l.
   d   Ventilation—the loss during respiration is greater in infants than in adults when compared with the body weight. The loss varies with the humidity.

    e Faecal loss is only a few ml per day.

    f Lactation—up to 900 ml per day.

The day-to-day fluctuation in the normal total body water amounts to up to ± 0.2 per cent of the body weight in 24 h in temperate climate with free access to fluids.

Dehydration

When water intake is restricted, there is transfer of water from the ICF to the ECF until the limit of possible transfer has been reached (i.e. body weight loss exceeds 10 per cent). The standard water deprivation test should be discontinued when the body weight has fallen by more than 5 per cent.

Overload

If excess water is retained, it is redistributed: 8 per cent in the vascular compartment, remainder in ISF and ICF. Oedema is not detectable until 4 litres have been retained in excess in the ECF.

WATER LOAD TEST

Oral 20 ml/kg body weight is given over 15–20 min (or i.v. as hypotonic glucose solution over a 45-min period). This represents 2 per cent of the body weight.

    Normal: 80 per cent of the load is excreted in 5 h with a minimal osmolality of 50 mosmol/kg H_2O of the urine.

    Abnormal

        Dehydration.

        Malabsorption.

        Abnormal water distribution

            Gross oedema.

            Gross ascites.

            Gross obesity.

            Dehydration.

            Congestive cardiac failure.

        Renal damage.

        Post-renal obstruction.

        Impaired adrenocortical function.

        True SIADH—inability to suppress ADH secretion, therefore less water excreted in 5 h ('reset osmostat'—80 per cent water load excreted in 5 h, but plasma sodium remains low).

Water Deprivation

Diabetes insipidus and related syndromes ⎫ continued urine
Diabetes mellitus   ⎬ output in spite of
Diuretics   ⎭ fluid deprivation.

Diurnal Urine Flow

In normal subjects there is a marked reduction in urine flow during sleep.

Reversal or Loss of Diurnal Variation in Urine Flow

Night-shift workers.
Oedema.
Renal failure.
Malabsorption.
Mineralocorticoid administration, Cushing's syndrome.
Addison's disease.
Hyperaldosteronism.
Head injury.

Diuresis

Water Diuresis

Increased water intake.
Insufficient ADH action
    Diabetes insipidus.
    Renal diabetes insipidus ⎫ failure to re-
    Renal tubular lesions   ⎬ spond to ADH
Chronic mineralocorticoid deficiency.
Hypokalaemia   ⎫ inability to produce
Hypercalcaemia ⎬ concentrated urine.
Drugs.

Osmotic Diuresis

Oral urea (30–60 g in 250 ml fluid) followed by diuresis with low urinary sodium concentration.
Hyperglycaemia
    Diabetic hyperglycaemia.
    Glucose infusion.
Mannose infusion.
Salt
    Excessive intake.

Abnormal loss
Response to diuretics.
Disease states.

Water Overload

see section Hydration and Toxicity, pp. 120–127.

2 Hydration and Tonicity of Body Fluids

Hypovolaemia
Hypervolaemia
Hyponatraemia
Hypernatraemia
Hyperosmolar
Dehydration and hyponatraemia
Normal hydration and
   hyponatraemia
Overhydration and hypotonicity
   (and SIADH)

Overhydration and
   normotonicity
Overhydration and hypertonicity
Normal hydration and
   hypertonicity
Dehydration and hypertonicity
Dehydration and isotonicity

   Maintenance of intracellular homeostasis, which is fundamental to cell life, depends on the maintenance of normal extracellular fluid (ECF) constitution, concentration and volume, with normal transfer of water and solute across cell membranes between the intracellular fluid (ICF) and the ECF. Alterations in the ECF affect the ICF and vice versa, and incidentally affect renal function and specific cell functions (e.g. osmoreceptors, respiratory centre cells, etc.).

   The ECF includes the circulation, with rapid transport of water and solutes around the body, which is separated from the cell membranes by the interstitial fluid (ISF). The circulatory volume is maintained as near normal as possible, for as long as possible in pathological states, overriding responses to changes in ECF osmolality, after certain limits of change have been exceeded.

   The normal individual will, on occasion, take in excess food and/or drink, markedly surplus to requirements, and on other occasions may suffer hunger and/or thirst, as a result of shortage of food and/or water. Body mechanisms maintain a steady state in the ECF and ICF for as long as possible during periods of excess or depletion. Following injury, protective mechanisms come into play, and these have been described as 'cave man responses'. In the absence of medical and/or surgical care, or even supplies of water and food, these responses include salt and water retention, increased coagulability of the blood with thrombocytosis, release of aldosterone, ADH, glucagon (with insulin supression, etc.). The injured man is thereby enabled to survive severe injury in

111

isolation for a few days, using his reservoirs of glycogen in the liver, then body fat and muscle protein in the absence of available food and water. The period of survival by these means is limited, and after a few days, the wounded man dies, or is fit enough to struggle out to scavenge for food and water once more.

These survival mechanisms are very important, as they automatically come into action after surgery (a specialized form of injury) and after accidental injury, even though surgical and medical treatment is available.

In terms of evolution and survival of the species, these protective mechanisms are important, but need to be remembered and considered during the treatment of patients, e.g. the persistence in the giving of intravenous fluid at the rate of 2–3 litres/day immediately after operation to ensure 'adequate urine flow' in patients (especially if elderly) is inviting potentially dangerous water retention and overload. Attempting to eliminate the water load, again, to establish 'adequate urine flow', often then results in very severe sudden hyponatraemia, if strong diuretics are given.

The laboratory results returned to clinicians only define the concentrations of sodium, potassium, chloride, bicarbonate, urea and creatinine in plasma (and urine). There is no laboratory test which gives a direct measure of body hydration (ranging from dehydration, through normal hydration, to overhydration). Body weight, allowing for the effects of any starvation, gives some measure of hydration change, when taken with the patient's history and physical examination. A rough estimation of plasma osmolality can be calculated from the plasma sodium, potassium, glucose and urea concentrations, and the actual plasma osmolality can be measured directly. A dehydrated patient with a low plasma sodium concentration has very different problems from an overhydrated patient with hyponatraemia, the abnormal state having been reached by different pathological pathways, resulting in different clinical states, eliciting different body responses and requiring different treatment. It is therefore very important that laboratory results are always read in the light of the clinical state and history of the patient. Normal results from the laboratory may be returned from samples from patients who may be overhydrated, normally hydrated or dehydrated, and these situations are shown in *Fig.* 1.

INTRODUCTION

Fig. 1 illustrates the various clinical syndromes in which hydration and tonicity are abnormally changed, with the normal state in the centre of the matrix. The description of signs and symptoms

HYPOTONICITY + DEHYDRATION (A)	HYPOTONICITY + NORMAL HYDRATION (B)	HYPOTONICITY + OVERHYDRATION (including SIADH) (C)
NORMAL TONICITY + DEHYDRATION (H)	NORMAL TONICITY + NORMAL HYDRATION (THE NORMAL STATE)	NORMAL TONICITY + OVERHYDRATION (D)
HYPERTONICITY + DEHYDRATION (G)	HYPERTONICITY + NORMAL HYDRATION (F)	HYPERTONICITY + OVERHYDRATION (E)

Fig. 1. Clinical variations in tonicity and hydration about the normal state. The capital letters A–H refer to descriptions of these various clinical states in the text.

found in pure dehydration, overhydration, hypertonicity and hypotonicity is to be read in the knowledge that any abnormal biochemical state is dynamic, with body defence mechanisms coming into action, and possibly the disease process which caused the biochemical abnormalities still active. The clinical states (A), (C), (E) and (G) are less transient than (B), (D), (F) and (H).

HYPOVOLAEMIA
Signs and Symptoms
These include those associated with the manner in which fluid is lost, e.g. vomiting, diabetes mellitus, etc., the effects of volume depletion, and the frequently associated electrolyte disturbances.

The signs and symptoms directly referable to hypovolaemia include:
Falling cardiac output, with falling blood pressure and rising pulse rate. The pulse becomes thready, tissue perfusion is reduced with peripheral vasoconstriction.
Progressive lassitude with easy fatiguability.
Thirst, unless suppressed by hyponatraemia, or disease process.
Muscle cramps.
Postural dizziness.
Abdominal pain (mesenteric ischaemia).
Chest pain (coronary ischaemia).
Confusion (cerebral ischaemia).
Hypotension and shock.
Progressive weight loss.
The increase in plasma urea is greater than increase in plasma creatinine—normal kidney response to effective circulatory volume depletion. If the rises in urea and creatinine are comparable, and urine sodium exceeds 20 mmol/l there is renal loss of salt and water.

Treatment

Water deficit can be calculated as

$$0.6 \times \text{body weight} \times \left(\frac{\text{Plasma sodium}}{140} - 1 \right)$$

The rate of fluid replacement should be at 50–100 ml/h in excess of the urine output plus the estimated insensible water loss plus any measured visible fluid loss, i.e. a positive fluid balance.

HYPERVOLAEMIA

Following excessive transfusion of blood into a normal subject, there is a transient rise in venous pressure, falling to normal when the transfusion is stopped. The extra blood is 'accommodated' in the lungs, veins and venous plexuses. The filling of the lungs results in a fall in vital capacity.

Continued transfusion with blood, plasma or isotonic saline is accompanied by sensations of fullness in the head and headache, tightness in the chest with dyspnoea. A dry cough develops, and moist râles can be heard at the lung bases. The jugular venous pressure is increased.

Bruising, petechiae and haemorrhages have been described after very large transfusions, but these are almost certainly due to dilution of the patient's platelets, rather than any volume effect.

Pitting oedema in an adult requires the accumulation of 3–4 litres excess of ECF, e.g. the unnecessary infusion of salt and water in excess of excretion, or intake of salt and water in the presence of renal failure.

HYPONATRAEMIA

Signs and Symptoms

Loss of appetite, followed by nausea and vomiting.
Abdominal pain.
Lightheadedness.
Increased cerebrospinal fluid pressure with papilloedema.
Weakness and lethargy.
Restlessness.
Confusion.
Delirium.
Psychosis.
Muscle twitches and tremor.
EEG abnormalities with epileptiform convulsions.

HYPEROSMOLAR STATES
Hypernatraemia
Signs and Symptoms
1 Lethargy progressing to coma.
2 Muscle rigidity, tremor and myoclonus may occur.
3 Spasticity and hyperreflexia.
4 Transient generalized chorea may progress to epileptiform convulsions.
5 Abnormal EEG readings.
6 Cerebrospinal fluid protein concentration is increased without pleocytosis.
7 Permanent brain damage may occur in infants suffering from rapidly developing hypernatraemia, who survive following treatment.

Hyperosmolar Syndrome
Signs and Symptoms
1 If the patient is conscious, he complains of extreme thirst unless there is hypothalamic damage with damage to the thirst centre.
2 Severe hyperpnoea.
3 Skin and mucous membranes are dry.
4 Confusion, stupor, coma, and rarely convulsions, with the most severe symptoms in the old and the very young.
5 Oliguria, unless there is also an osmotic diuresis.
6 Whole blood haemoglobin and haematocrit are increased with increased plasma protein concentration.
7 Water is lost from all the fluid spaces in the body.
  A 20 per cent increase in plasma sodium equals a 20 per cent loss of body water.

A. DEHYDRATION WITH HYPONATRAEMIA
Causes
Simple Classification
1 Initial isotonic dehydration with contraction of the ECF, followed by partial replacement by water and/or hypotonic fluid.
2 Salt loss in excess of water loss.
3 Any potassium depletion increases the rate of loss of sodium.

Practical Classification
1. *Gastrointestinal fluid loss* (urine sodium < 20 mmol/l)
Up to 3 litres of fluid containing approx. 140 mmol/l sodium and 10–20 mmol/l potassium. Gastric and small intestinal fluids tend to be isotonic, with potassium 10–20 mmol/l.

a *Saliva loss*: Hypotonic fluid 20 mmol/l cation. With increasing saliva loss, the saliva tends to become isotonic.

b *Nasogastric aspiration*: Gastric fluid is isotonic.

c *Oesophageal obstruction.*

d *Pyloric obstruction*: With vomiting more water than solute is lost.

e *Acute gastric dilatation*: Up to 5 litres (30 per cent of ECF) may be 'trapped'.

f *Intestinal obstruction*: Fluid passes into gut lumen.

g *Gastrointestinal fistulae.*

h *Ileostomy malfunction*: A well-functioning established ileostomy excretes hypotonic fluid.

i *Diarrhoea*: Moderate diarrhoea—up to 3 litres per day.

         Severe pseudomembranous colitis } 1 litre per hour
         Cholera   can be lost.

Stools are normally hypotonic, containing 20 mmol/l cations. With increasing rate of loss, the concentration approaches isotonicity (but not in babies).

2. *'Third space' losses* (urine sodium < 20 mmol/l)

a Burns
Pancreatitis.
Muscle trauma, severe limb trauma.
Peritonitis.

b Haemorrhage }
Plasma loss } fluid replacement without sodium replacement.

c Massive sweat loss with water replacement only.

3. *Renal losses* (urine sodium > 20 mmol/l)

a Excessive diuretic therapy with access to unlimited water.

b Mineralocorticoid deficiency.

c Sodium-losing nephritis.

d Renal proximal tubule acidosis (Type II)—obligatory loss of sodium and bicarbonate in the urine.

e Nephrocalcinosis.

f Severe metabolic alkalosis—obligatory loss of sodium and bicarbonate in the urine.

g Osmotic diuresis—glucose
                   —urea   } obligatory loss of sodium and
                   —mannitol } bicarbonate in the urine.

h Patients with:
—nephrocalcinosis
—polycystic renal disease   when put on low-sodium diet,
—medullary cystic disease   develop volume contraction
  of kidney   with hyponatremia, as they
—other tubulo-interstitial   are unable to retain sodium.
  renal disease

N.B. The body breaks down body fat, so that 1 g fat gives 1 ml of water without salt. Similarly muscle breakdown releases protein, and 1 g of protein gives 1 ml of water plus potassium, but virtually no sodium.

Signs and Symptoms

The severity is proportional to the rate of development of change from normal, and the degree of change. Older patients may give a false impression of dehydration, as they have lost subcutaneous fat, and their skin is losing its elasticity; the weight of such patients may be very useful.

Thready pulse
Tachycardia
Falling blood pressure
Low CVP
Reduced eyeball tension
Dry mouth
Dry skin and mucous membranes
Sunken cheeks, with reduced skin elasticity
Furred tongue
Longitudinal wrinkling of the tongue
Weight loss
   Mild—2–5 per cent of body weight lost.
   Moderate—5–10 per cent of body weight lost.
   Severe—more than 10 per cent of body weight lost.
Acute weight loss suggests fluid loss (i.e. in excess of 300 g/day). Calorie-lack weight loss = 150–300 g per day—rarely up to 500 g per day.
Oliguria
Thirst—suggests EAV reduced $\Big\}$ nausea follows later.
   —suggests hyperosmolality
Disorientation progressing through delirium to coma, fits, and finally death.

Laboratory Findings

Reduced urine volume with sp. gr. 1·020–1·040 (1200–1400 mosmol/l) unless there is also renal disease. Urine sodium low, unless there is renal disease or adrenocortical insufficiency, congenital adrenal hyperplasia, inappropriate tapering off of steroids.
Plasma sodium low.
Plasma urea, creatinine and uric acid increased. Plasma protein increased. (Urea > creatinine later.)

Whole blood haematocrit increased (each rise of 0·1 (1 per cent) is equivalent to the loss of 500 ml fluid—100 ml from ECF, 400 ml from ISF).

Physiopathology

The renin–angiotensin system is stimulated, resulting in vasoconstriction. Aldosterone release is stimulated by falling plasma sodium, and results in sodium retention.

Falling plasma osmolality leads to ADH release, which makes the distal renal tubules permeable to water, and water is retained, with concentration of the urine. ADH release occurs in response to the fall in fluid volume, regardless of the fluid tonicity in the body. With increasing hypotonicity of the ECF water enters the cells (ICF), and the ECF is further shrunken. Each litre of extra water lowers the plasma sodium by 3 mmol/l. There is loss of intracellular anions leading to intercellular hypo-osmolality.

A patient with low plasma sodium and urine sodium exceeding 20 mmol/l:

1 Not on diuretics,
2 Not receiving extra salt,
   suggests:
      adrenal insufficiency with aldosterone lack.
      recovery phase after acute renal tubule necrosis.
      recovery phase after relief of urinary tract obstruction.
      brain injury or infection—leading to 'salt wasting'.

Treatment

Sodium deficit in mmol =

$$(140 - \text{patient's plasma sodium in mmol/l}) \times \frac{\text{Body weight (kg)}}{2}.$$

For every 0·1 (1 per cent) of haematocrit above normal, allow 500 ml, correcting over 48 h. 'Safe' replacement = calculated deficit in mmol × 1 in ECF. With satisfactory treatment the urine flow should reach 50 ml/min and eventually normal body weight is regained, allowing for calorie loss due to starvation, with attainment of normal haematocrit.

Volume deficits can be replaced relatively rapidly (i.e. over 24–48 h). It the patient is in shock and dehydration with a very large fluid deficit, infuse 1 litre of isotonic saline each 30 min until the urine flow reaches 50 ml/min, monitoring the CVP which should be kept below 15 mmHg. Correct up to a plasma sodium of 120 mmol/l.

Correction of tonicity and/or acid–base disorders must be corrected more slowly. Treatment should be with isotonic saline or isotonic modified buffered saline. Gastric aspirate can be replaced volume for volume with 0·45 per cent NaCl plus 40 mmol K added per litre, Gastrointestinal fluid loss can be replaced volume for volume with: Na 140; Cl 100; HCO_3 precursors 40; KCl 40 mmol/l (Na 140, lactate 25, K20).

Daily fluid allotment (approx. 2·5 litre) plus replacement of previous 24 h fluid loss (adjust every 12 h if the losses are excessive). Very severe hyponatraemia induced by excessive thiazide therapy (e.g. plasma sodium <100 mmol/l) has been treated by peritoneal dialysis, or haemodialysis using a dialysate containing glucose 75·6 mmol/l, sodium 140 mmol/l and potassium 4·4 mmol/l to raise plasma sodium at 0·83 mmol/h to more than 120 mmol/l.

B. HYPOTONICITY WITH NORMAL HYDRATION

Causes

Acute

Acute increased water intake in:

 a Patients developing acute hypovolaemia, e.g. haemorrhage.
 b During treatment with strong diuretics.
 c During the first 48 hours after surgical operation or trauma, especially in the elderly.
 d In any patient with impairment of water excretion, e.g. renal damage.

2. *Less Rapid, and Chronic*

 a Coincidental exact replacement of ECF loss with water and/or hypotonic saline.
 b 'Reset osmostat'. Patients who have maintained a normal ECF volume in a hypo-osmolar state, may have 'reset' their osmoreceptors, with control at a new level outside the normal range.
 c Glucocorticoid deficiency
    i   Anterior hypopituitarism.
    ii Hypoadrenocortical function.
    iii Sudden cessation of glucocorticoid therapy.
 d Hypothyroidism.
 e Some patients treated with diuretics, with potassium depletion.
 f Physical stress, emotional stress, with thirst (?).
 g Antidiuretic drugs
    stimulating ADH release;
    potentiating ADH action;

e.g. chlorpropamide causing increased ADH release plus sensitization of the renal collecting ducts to the action of ADH.
ADH-like hormone produced by malignant tumour.

h Polydipsia with vomiting.

i SIADH.

Signs and Symptoms

When there is a rapid fall in plasma sodium concentration from, say, 140 mmol/l to 130 mmol/l with normal total body fluid, within a few minutes to an hour, e.g. acute water intoxication:

1. The patient complains of feeling bloated, a 'fullness in the head', headache and anorexia.

2. Nausea develops, occasionally with actual vomiting.

3. Muscle cramps occur.

4. With more severe changes in tonicity, the patient becomes lethargic, and disorientated. Fits may occur.

5. There may be altered level of consciousness.

6. Papilloedema develops, and there are signs of increased intracranial pressure.

7. The deep tendon reflexes become abnormal. The progressive severity of signs and symptoms develop as the state of hypervolaemia with hypotonicity develops (C).

Laboratory Findings

Urine sodium concentration is greater than 20 mmol/l in the absence of diuretic therapy, unless there has been restriction of sodium intake, when the urine sodium concentration falls.

Treatment

Treat the cause.

C. OVERHYDRATION WITH HYPOTONICITY (INCLUDING SIADH)

Causes

1. Increased water load.
2. Decreased water clearance.
3. Combination of (1) and (2).

Signs and Symptoms

Signs and symptoms are proportional to the rate of development of hypotonicity and water retention. Patients complain of fatigue and apprehension. Muscle weakness with abdominal cramps develop. There may be diarrhoea and oliguria progressing to anuria. Oedema increases and convulsions occur.

Laboratory Findings

Plasma sodium concentrations are low, e.g. 110 mmol/l. (140–110) = 30 mmol/l, and each 3 mmol/l of sodium reduction is equivalent to 1 litre of water retained. Thus this low plasma sodium, in the absence of sodium deficiency, represents 10 litres of water evenly distributed between the ECF and the ICF.

Pathophysiology of Hyponatraemia with Overhydration

1 ECF increased.
2 ICF increased.
3 Effective blood volume reduced.
4 AVP variable.
5 Urine sodium output reduced.
6 Plasma renin activity reduced,
    i.e. the kidney acts as though it is persistently underperfused.

Excessive Fluid Intake with Retention
Hypotonic Overhydration, Fluid Expansion with Hypotonicity, Water Intoxication

Administration of 5 per cent dextrose solution, or dextrose-saline solution in the 48 h period immediately after surgery or trauma.
Overload with 10 per cent glucose in 0·18 per cent saline during labour causes hyponatraemic water overload in mother and newborn infant (1200 ml/day only required).
    Polydipsia
    Psychogenic (uncommon).
    Beer 'binge' (common); plasma sodium may fall below 130 mmol/l for short periods during a heavy drinking bout.
    Baby given excess water, e.g. in the 'treatment' of cow's milk intolerance.
    In the normal subject, if water intake exceeds 36 litres in 24 h, plasma sodium concentration falls, as the renal excretion rate of free water is exceeded (if the normal protective mechanism of vomiting does not come into effect).
    Salt depletion with increased water intake.
    Diuretic therapy with plentiful water intake.
    Cirrhosis of the liver ⎱ dilutional hyponatremia occurs with a
    Renal disease   ⎰   lower daily intake of fluid.
    Mannitol infusion.

Starvation Hyponatraemia (pre- and post-surgery or trauma)

After 15 per cent loss of body weight, dilutional hypotonicity develops. One gram of fat releases 1 ml of water on oxidation, and 1 g of muscle releases 1 ml of water plus potassium. Any weight gain associated with water retention is masked by calorie loss. A postoperative patient will lose about 300 g per day if he is not eating, but taking fluids.

Urine sodium concentration of less than 20 mmol/l in the absence of diuretic therapy is found in:

1. Congestive cardiac failure (low cardiac output with low renal blood flow). (There may be an underlying magnesium deficit, and magnesium supplements may be useful.)

2. Cirrhosis of the liver (low plasma albumin with low oncotic pressure; sequestration of ECF in ascitic fluid).

3. Nephrosis (low plasma albumin with low oncotic pressure; and sequestration of ECF in ISF oedema fluid).

Baroreceptor stimulation results in release of ADH, with decreased distal renal fluid tubule delivery, which results from the reduced glomerular filtration rate, increased proximal tubule fluid reabsorption, plus ADH-induced distal tubule fluid reabsorption.

Following trauma and/or surgery, organic solutes escape from cells, bringing water into the ECF, and potassium, magnesium and phosphate are lost in the urine. In its extreme form this used to be described as the 'sick cell syndrome', when it was postulated that hydrogen ions and sodium ions entered the cells.

Stress, surgery and other injuries all result in the release of both ADH and aldosterone, with resulting salt and water retention (a primitive body defence mechanism).

Acute and Chronic Renal Failure

The urine sodium output exceeds 20 mmol/l and with the reduced effective renal mass, water overload easily occurs. When the GFR is down to 5 ml/min, amounting to a total filtrate of 7·2 litre per day, only 1·5 litre of that is free water per day, which can be generated and excreted. Overload is therefore all too easy. Peritoneal dialysis of renal patients with solutions with too weak sodium concentration have caused dilutional hyponatraemia.

Hyponatraemia with Overhydration and Impaired Water Excretion

1. Primary and secondary adrenal glucocorticoid deficiency. There is impaired ability to excrete a water load, which is corrected by glucocorticoid. (The abnormality is not related to AVP (ADH) action, renal blood flow or to the GFR.

2. Chlorpropamide.
3. Myxoedema. There is reduction in GFR plus reduced medullary blood flow.

Extra fluid is held in the ECF in:
1. Oedema fluid.
2. Ascites.
3. Large effusions.
4. 'Third space', e.g. *a.* Paralytic ileus; *b.* Severe peritonitis.

Hypo-osmolar States associated with Increased ADH Release

1. **Stimulation of ADH Release**
   a Hypotension, hypovolaemia, secondary to blood loss or reduction in ECF.
   b Reduced cardiac output leading to increased proximal tubule reabsorption of salt and water from glomerular filtrate
      i Congestive cardiac failure.
      ii Nephrosis with reduced plasma albumin and hypovolaemia.
      iii Cirrhosis with ascites, or after rapid paracentesis.
      iv Post-mitral valvotomy, with relief of distension of left atrial receptors.
   c Response to pain, nausea.

2. **Inappropriate Release of ADH** (*see below*)

C. SYNDROME OF INAPPROPRIATE ADH RELEASE (SIADH)

Causes

1. **Ectopic Production of ADH or ADH-like Substance**
   Lung tumours (35 per cent of all oat-cell carcinomas).
   Bronchial carcinoid.
   Pancreatic carcinoma.
   Other carcinomas less common.

2. **ADH from Posterior Pituitary**
   a Inappropriate ADH administration.
   b *Enhanced release of ADH*
   Cerebral neoplasm ⎫
   Intracranial trauma ⎪ disturbance of hypothalamus or
   Intracranial infection ⎬ posterior pituitary resulting
   Intracranial surgery ⎭ in release of ADH.

Drugs
Clofibrate.
Vincristine.
Carbamazepine.
Nicotine.

3. *Abnormal AVP Response to Volume Receptors*

a. Congestive cardiac failure. Proximal renal tubule retention of sodium and water, urine sodium less than 10–15 mmol/l, urine osmolality 350–400 mosmol/l. This results in greater passive back diffusion of water from the collecting ducts. Excessive release of ADH leads to low RPF and low GFR, with inability to produce concentrated urine. ECV is diminished, and the kidneys behave as though they were underperfused. With decreased delivery of sodium to the loop of Henle, there is dissipation of the normal medullary osmotic gradient.

b. Cirrhosis. Similar excessive reabsorption of sodium and water from the proximal renal tubules. The colloid osmotic pressure is low, with reduced plasma albumin, and the kidneys behave as though they were underperfused.

c. Nephrosis. There is excessive sodium and water reabsorption in the proximal renal tubules. diminished ECV results in the kidneys responding as though they are underperfused. The colloid osmotic pressure is lower than normal, as plasma albumin concentration is low.

d. Positive-pressure respiration. Intermittent positive-pressure respiration using a ventilator causes release of ADH by stimulating thoracic receptors.

e. Lung disease
 i Asthma
 ii Pneumonia
 iii Pulmonary
    tuberculosis
} Increased intrathoracic pressure results in reduced venous return to the heart, and 'appropriate' release of ADH.

f. Hypothyroidism.

g. Hypoadrenalism—limitation of effective blood volume results in release of excess inappropriate ADH.

h. Guillain–Barré syndrome—hypotonia results in reduced venous return and 'osmostat resetting'.

4. *Enhanced Renal Tubule Response to Normal Levels of ADH (AVP)*

Response to drug therapy:
a Carbamazepine.
b Chlorpropamide.
c Hydrochlorothiazide.

d Hydroflumethazide.
e Cyclothiazide.

Alternative Classification of SIADH

1. Group of patients with erratic and apparently independent osmoreceptor function.
2. Qualitatively normal response to increasing plasma tonicity, but 'reset' at below 275 mosmol/kg (the normal lower limit).
3. Persistent elevated plasma ADH in face of plasma hypotonicity:
   Meningitis ⎱
   Skull fracture ⎰ hypothalamic stimulation.
   Ectopic tumour production.
4. Smallest clinical group (10 per cent)—vasopressin suppressed in hypotonicity and does not increase normally above physiological levels:
   Vasopressin-independent urine diluting defect.
   Enhanced sensitivity to vasopressin.

Pathophysiology

Moderate increase in intravascular volume results in increased RPF and GFR, leading to reduced distal tubule sodium reabsorption.

Volume expansion results in suppression of aldosterone secretion, i.e. patients in negative sodium balance with inappropriately concentrated urine.

Hyponatraemia—plasma sodium less than 130 mmol/l.

Hypo-osmolality of plasma.

Intracellular potassium depletion develops.

Continued renal sodium excretion, more than 30 mmol/l with intake equalling output. Urine tonicity is higher than expected for plasma osmolality or fluid ingestion.

Absence of body fluid depletion (water retention occurs). Normal skin turgor and normal blood pressure.

Adrenal function normal.

Renal function normal, other than the inability to form a dilute urine, secondary to inappropriate ADH release. Plasma AVP > 510 pg/ml (normal = 2–10 pg/ml).

Severity of signs and symptoms

Proportional to depression of plasma sodium.

   Proportional to water retention (several litres).

   Proportional to rate of development—can develop rapidly in children.

Experimentally, when Excess Water and ADH are given to Normal Subjects

1. Retention of water, leading to increased body fluid volume with hyponatraemia and hypotonicity of plasma, without oedema (fluid retained in intravascular fluid, ECF and ICF).
2. GFR increases with increased filtered sodium load.
3. Aldosterone secretion suppressed, with increased sodium load filtered by renal tubules.
4. Urine sodium excretion continues in spite of hyponatraemia.
5. Proximal tubular reabsorption of sodium and water decreased.

When a patient suffering from SIADH is deprived of water, correction of the plasma sodium level occurs with insensible water loss. On an average-normal sodium intake with expanded fluid volume, there is no loss of additional sodium. On a very low sodium intake there may be no increase in sodium excretion.

The patient may excrete a urine more dilute than plasma filtrate, but it is not maximally dilute, i.e. loss of 'free water' by insensible loss plus urine is less than the intake of 'free water'.

There may be other renal faults which do not prevent the development of SIADH, e.g. renal tubular acidosis.

After oral or intravenous alcohol:

a. Water diuresis with rise in plasma sodium = endogenous ADH causing SIADH.

b. No response suggests ectopic ADH from tumour.

(Diphenylhydantoin also suppresses ADH with an action similar to alcohol.)

Treatment of SIADH

1   Treat cause, if possible.
2   Treatment of symptomatic hypo-osmolality with hyperhydration:
    Slow—reduce water intake.
    Acute—water restriction; demeclocycline, up to 300 mg t.d.s. (if urine osmolality > 900 mosmol/Kg) (avoid if there is renal damage, care if liver damage). Biological half-life = 16 h. Effective plasma level may persist for 24–48 h, acting on distal renal tubules, blocking the action of ADH. Fludrocortisone, 0·1 mg on alternate days (replacement steroid and cortisol in Addison's adrenal failure; replacement of steroid in adrenal hyperplasia with congenital salt loss).

Acute Emergency Treatment

Frusemide bolus 40–60 mg i.v. When the urine diuresis starts, give 3–5 per cent saline i.v. at the rate of 200 ml/h, giving up to 500 ml only.

Check potassium level in plasma, and replace if falling below normal. Continue with water restriction, demeclocycline plus fludrocortisone, as above.

Oral urea 30–60 g/day in 1–2 litres flavoured water orally daily with access to water—the urine output of sodium and urea are inversely related. ADH increases water and urea permeability of collecting ducts, with increased urea trapping in medulla. This increases passive water extraction in the thin descending limb of the proximal tubule, with resulting increased salt concentration in the thin descending limb which is selectively permeable to sodium chloride. The low blood urea concentration found in SIADH leads to difficulty in withholding the sodium load. ? abnormal loss of urea in SIADH.

D. NORMOTONICITY WITH OVERHYDRATION
Signs and Symptoms
As in 'hypervolaemia', e.g. bounding pulse, etc.

Causes
1. Iatrogenic
Sudden expansion of the ECF with isotonic fluid. Overtransfusion with isotonic saline.

2. Pathological
Sudden onset of cardiac failure in a previously healthy patient.

E. HYPERTONICITY WITH OVERHYDRATION
Signs and Symptoms
1 Acute weight gain.
2 Pitting oedema. Oedema of the tissues may be noted during surgery.
3 Dyspnoea with moist râles.
4 Puffy eyelids.
5 Bounding pulse.
6 Possible consequences
   a Cerebral bleeding.
   b Pulmonary oedema.
   c Systemic hypertension.

Causes
Iatrogenic or accidental excessive replacement of fluid losses with isotonic or hypertonic fluids, with loss of water from lungs and skin.

F. HYPERTONICITY WITH NORMAL HYDRATION
Causes

1. Coincidental replacement of fluid loss with hypertonic fluids, e.g. replacement with isotonic saline without making allowance for water lost in sweat and respiration.

2. Occasional central nervous system lesions, especially in the region of the posterior fossa, resulting in temporary ?'osmostat reset'. The plasma sodium concentration may be maintained at 160 mmol/l in spite of salt restriction and increased fluid intake:

    a   Lesion causes thirst mechanism defect.
    b   Lesion results in insensitivity of osmoreceptors.
    c   (*a*) + (*b*).

After a water load, plasma osmolality approaches normality in (*a*), but the water load is ineffective in (*b*). Chlorpropamide relieves the hypernatraemia in (*b*).

G. HYPERTONICITY WITH DEHYDRATION
(Dehydration, hypertonic dehydration, hyperosmolar dehydration)

Causes

1. *Lack of Fluid Intake* (with continuing output)

Patient restrained from drinking, or anorexia.
Comatose patient.
Baby given concentrated feeds.
Adult tube feeds, e.g. neurosurgery hyperalimentation.
Uraemia with raised blood urea.
Normal adult
    In desert without water.
    At sea without water.

2. *Water Loss*

Loss from skin and lungs—increased by high fever. The lung is the only site from which water can be lost without loss of sodium.
Hyperventilation.
Gastrointestinal tract
    Rapid loss of saliva (rare)
    Rapid loss of large volumes of fluid   }   the fluid lost is
        from colon   initially hypotonic.

3. *Loss of Ability to Concentrate Urine*
Renal Diuresis

Diuretics in excess.

Uncontrolled diabetes mellitus.
Hyperalimentation with glucose, resulting in a glucose-induced diuresis.
Diabetes insipidus
  Pituitary—10–20 litres of urine per day. Patient can manage until fluid intake restricted.
  Nephrogenic—7–8 litres of urine per day.
  (penthrane anaesthesia).
Post-acute renal tubule necrosis recovery.
Post-renal obstruction relief recovery, followed by diuresis.

4. Following Infusion Therapy
Isotonic saline given to replace water loss.
Hypertonic saline infusion with low fluid intake and continued water loss from lungs.
Infusion of 5 per cent sodium bicarbonate after cardiac arrest.
Peritoneal dialysis using too high concentrations of sodium and glucose (water is removed from the ECF faster than sodium is removed).

5. Hyperosmolality in Cells with Normal Plasma Sodium Concentration and Hyperosmolality of Plasma
Diabetic ketoacidosis—plasma sodium falls by 1·5 mmol/l per increase in 5·6 mmol/l glucose. N.B. Beware of false sodium readings associated with massive hyperlipidaemia.
Hypertonic mannitol infusion resulting in diuresis.
Peritoneal dialysis with hypertonic glucose solution.
Diabetic hyperosmolar non-ketotic acidosis.

Signs and Symptoms
The signs and symptoms are proportional to the degree of change, and to the rate of development of change. Thirst is severe. The mouth is dry, with a furred tongue, and the mucous membranes are dry. The skin is flushed with loss of elasticity. Eyeball tension is lost, and tears are absent. In an adult shock develops when 10 litres of body fluid have been lost. Infants and children can lose 10–15 per cent of their body weight before dehydration is obvious (in the absence of serial weighing). In infants the anterior fontanelle is depressed.
Urine volume is greatly reduced, until anuria occurs. It is important to remember that infants are unable to concentrate urine to the same degree as adults. In infants the earlier symptoms of irritability are replaced by lethargy, then coma with seizures.

Brain cells are very sensitive to hypertonic dehydration, and infants under 2 years of age fed concentrated feeds may develop brain haemorrhages.

EEG readings are abnormal.

Plasma osmolality increases progressively, and death occurs in adults when 14 litres of the total body fluid have been lost.

Laboratory Findings

Plasma sodium exceeds 145 mmol/l (may exceed 160 mmol/l). Plasma osmolality may exceed 350 mosmol/l. Plasma sodium rises by 3 mmol/l for every litre of body water lost. Urine findings depend on the cause of hypertonic dehydration and its clinical course. Whole blood haematocrit rises by 0·1 (1 per cent) for each 500 ml of ECF water lost (100 ml plasma water plus 400 ml ISF). Urine urea concentration rises with reduced urine sodium excretion.

Mild Dehydration

Five per cent of body weight lost, with body fluids still isotonic.

Moderate Dehydration

Ten per cent of body weight lost. Urine concentration greater than 800 mosmol/l (sp. gr. 1·025), except in infants. Plasma sodium may rise, with falling plasma pH. The transfer of water from the ICF to the ECF is at its limit.

Severe Dehydration

Very severe pathological state with low blood pressure, rapid and weak pulse. Plasma urea, potassium and phosphate are all increased, with plasma pH 7·1–6·8 (80–160 nmol/l). At this stage the mortality rate is high. The glomerular filtration rate must be severely reduced in otherwise normal patients before phosphate is retained.

Physiopathology

Osmoreceptors affected by increases in osmolality exceeding 2 per cent stimulate ADH release; baroreceptors in the carotid arch are less sensitive and respond when the decrease in blood pressure is more than 10 per cent by stimulating ADH release.

ADH release results in distal tubular sodium reabsorption, but ultimately maintenance of the circulatory volume takes precedence over control of osmolality.

If the blood volume falls with a raised plasma sodium, this is followed by falling blood pressure and falling glomerular filtration rate, and rising blood urea.

A rapid rise in plasma sodium leads to cellular shrinkage in the brain, with tearing of the smaller blood vessels and consequent brain damage. This is more likely to occur in infants and may occur in infants under 2 years old, when they are fed with concentrated feeds, with consequent inability to excrete excess solute. The EEG is abnormal, and stuporose infants lapse into coma with high plasma osmolality.

Muscle and other body cells adapt to hyperosmolar states by loss of water and a gain in intracellular cations. The brain in some circumstances can protect itself from the effects of hyperosmolar states by the *de novo* generation of solute in the brain cells ('idiogenic osmols').

Treatment

The rate of return to normal values is very important, and should be slow to allow a slow steady change in osmolality over a period of at least 2–3 days, using 0·45 per cent saline plus glucose. The plasma sodium should not fall faster than 15 mmol/l per 4 h. Whenever possible, water replacement should be by mouth. Obviously specific causes of hypertonic dehydration must be treated.

Possibly 8–10 mg dexamethasone should be given intravenously stat, followed by 4–6 mg 12 hourly during the first 2 days of replacement therapy. Seizures, if they occur, should be controlled by diazepam, and the rate of replacement slowed down. Too rapid replacement is associated with a risk of congestive cardiac failure and oedema.

H. DEHYDRATION WITH ISOTONICITY

Causes

Found for a short period during treatment of dehydration with hypertonicity.   Coincidence of urine concentration such that body isotonicity is maintained, with loss of water from respiration and sweating.

Gastrointestinal fluid loss with coincidental replacement to maintain isotonicity.

Aspiration of (*a*) pleural fluid; (*b*) ascitic fluid.

With dehydration, fluid will move across cell membranes in an attempt to maintain the effective arterial volume. This state is unstable and will rapidly change from day to day.

3 Disorders of Hydrogen Ion Concentration; Metabolic/Respiratory Acidosis/Alkalosis; Mixed Disorders

Disturbances of hydrogen ion concentration
Non-respiratory acidosis
Respiratory acidosis
Metabolic alkalosis
Respiratory alkalosis
Combined metabolic and respiratory disorders
   Respiratory acidosis and respiratory alkalosis
   Respiratory acidosis, acute and chronic
   Metabolic acidosis and respiratory acidosis
   Respiratory acidosis and metabolic alkalosis
   Respiratory alkalosis and metabolic alkalosis
   Metabolic acidosis and respiratory alkalosis
   Metabolic acidosis and metabolic alkalosis

METABOLIC/RESPIRATORY ALKALOSIS/ACIDOSIS
(Hydrogen ion concentration changes)

When plasma hydrogen ion concentration is expressed in pH units, the limits of change which can be tolerated by the body appear to be smaller than when expressed as nmol/l (*Fig. 2*). Using quoted extreme limits compatible with short-term survival, plasma hydrogen ion concentration can vary by a factor of 10 (15–150 nmol/l approx.) but this only appears as pH 6·8–7·8 (7·8 represents an increase of +15 per cent on 6·8).

The normal subject manages to maintain his plasma hydrogen ion concentration within a very small range. In venous blood the normal range is 48–40 nmol/l (pH 7·32–7·40), and in arterial blood the normal range is 44–36 nmol/l (pH 7·36–7·44), very small when compared with the extremes possible in pathological states.

Protection from rapid extreme changes in hydrogen ion concentration occurs as a result of:

a. 'Mopping up' of hydrogen ions by buffer systems.

b. Rapid changes in rate of excretion of carbon dioxide in exhaled breath, and hence hydrogen ion concentration via bicarbonate formation/breakdown.

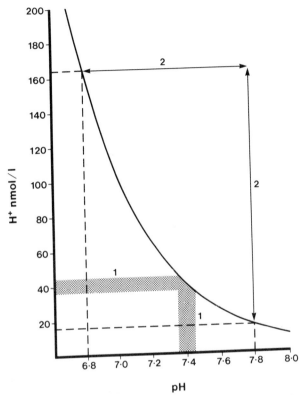

Fig. 2. Comparison of hydrogen ion concentration (nmol/l) and pH in plasma. 1, Shaded area = normal plasma range. 2, Extreme limits compatible with life.

c. Less rapid renal regulation of hydrogen ion excretion via the kidney. The kidneys eliminate 60 mmol hydrogen ions per day, and the urine hydrogen ion concentration can normally range from approximately 31 000 to 16 nmol/l (i.e. × approx. 2000) (pH 4·5–7·8).

There is greater potential for change in plasma hydrogen ion concentration from 44 to 160 nmol/l (pH 7·36–6·8) representing a four-fold increase in hydrogen ion concentration, than from 36 to 16 nmol/l (pH 7·44–7·8) representing a halving of hydrogen ion concentration. This reflects the normal continuous generation of hydrogen ions during body metabolism. Formation of hydroxyl ions with increase in pH above normal (fall in hydrogen ion concentration) is very unusual, and probably never occurs in man.

This section describes the various clinical conditions of metabolism (respiratory/metabolic acidosis/alkalosis (*Fig.* 3)) and clinical states combining metabolic and respiratory acidosis and/or alkalosis (*Fig.* 4).

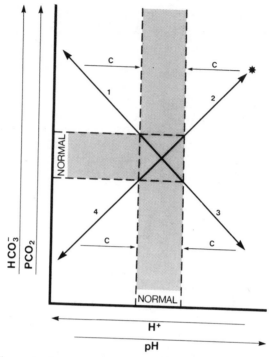

Fig. 3. Changes in plasma pH (or hydrogen ion concentration) in: 1, Respiratory acidosis (primary increase in P_{CO_2}). 2, Non-respiratory alkalosis (primary increase in HCO_3^-). * Unusual for P_{CO_2} to exceed 7·1 kPa (60 mmHg). 3, Respiratory alkalosis (primary decrease in P_{CO_2}). 4, Non-respiratory acidosis (primary decrease in HCO_3^-). c = direction of compensation, i.e. approaching normal pH (or hydrogen ion concentration).

DISTURBANCES OF HYDROGEN ION CONCENTRATION

The plasma pH depends on the bicarbonate buffer system, with its pK of 6·1 and the $\log_{10}$ of the ratio of plasma bicarbonate/carbon dioxide, which is normally the $\log_{10}$ of 20:

$$pH = pK + \log\frac{(\text{Bicarbonate under metabolic control})}{(CO_2 \text{ under respiratory control})}$$
$$= 6·1 + \log 20$$
$$= 6·1 + 1·3$$
$$= 7·4$$

Two hundred ml of CO_2 are produced at rest every minute— potentially 13 000 mmol carbonic acid per day.

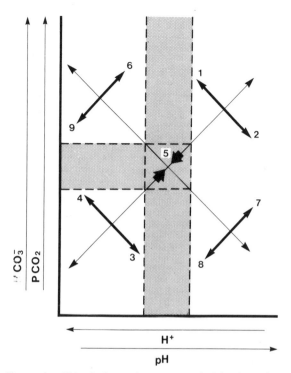

Fig. 4. Changes in pH (or hydrogen ion concentration) in plasma in combined metabolic and respiratory disorders: 1, Metabolic alkalosis complicated by respiratory acidosis. 2, Metabolic alkalosis complicated by respiratory alkalosis. 3, Metabolic acidosis complicated by respiratory alkalosis. 4, Metabolic acidosis complicated by respiratory acidosis. 5, Metabolic acidosis and metabolic alkalosis. 6, Respiratory acidosis complicated by metabolic alkalosis. 7, Respiratory alkalosis complicated by metabolic alkalosis, 8, Respiratory alkalosis complicated by metabolic acidosis. 9, Respiratory acidosis complicated by metabolic acidosis. 1, 3, 5, 6 and 8 'compensating' towards normal pH; 2, 4, 7 and 9 compounding abnormality of pH.

But only 1/800 is converted to carbonic acid, and 799/800 is carried as CO_2 in the plasma and ISF.

$$CO_2 + H_2O \rightleftharpoons H_2CO_3 \rightleftharpoons HCO_3^- + H^+.$$

One in each 1000 of the molecules of carbonic acid ionize, and there are 20 molecules of HCO_3^- per molecule of carbonic acid, H_2CO_3.

Normal plasma HCO_3^- concentration is approximately 24 mmol/l, and the corresponding $P{CO_2}$ is approximately 1·2 mmol/l (40 mmHg). The concentration of CO_2 is approximately 300 times the concentration of H_2CO_3.

Using the equation $pH = pK + \log$ (bicarbonate$/P_{CO_2}$) it is possible to define metabolic acidosis and alkalosis, and respiratory acidosis and alkalosis in simple terms.

Metabolic Alkalosis

$$pH = pK + \log\frac{\text{(Primary increase in bicarbonate)}}{\text{(Later secondary compensatory rise in } P_{CO_2})}.$$

The plasma pH tends to rise with increasing plasma bicarbonate. Plasma P_{CO_2} rises later, and to a lesser extent, so that the ratio Bicarbonate$/CO_2$ is more than 20.

Metabolic Acidosis

$$pH = pK + \log\frac{\text{(Primary decrease in bicarbonate)}}{\text{(Later secondary compensatory fall in } P_{CO_2})}.$$

The plasma pH tends to fall with the falling bicarbonate, and the plasma P_{CO_2} falls later and to a lesser extent, so that the ratio Bicarbonate$/CO_2$ is less than 20.

Respiratory Alkalosis

$$pH = pK + \log\frac{\text{(Secondary decrease in bicarbonate)}}{\text{(Primary decrease in } P_{CO_2})}.$$

The plasma pH tends to rise with falling P_{CO_2}. The plasma bicarbonate also falls, but later, and to a lesser extent, so that the Bicarbonate$/CO_2$ ratio is more than 20.

Respiratory Acidosis

$$pH = pK + \log\frac{\text{(Secondary increase in bicarbonate)}}{\text{(Primary increase in } P_{CO_2})}.$$

The plasma pH tends to fall with increasing P_{CO_2}. The plasma bicarbonate also rises, but later and to a lesser extent, so that the Bicarbonate$/CO_2$ ratio is less than 20.

In normal subjects severe exercise results in a CO_2 production rate ten times the resting rate. Increased ventilation with faster and deeper breathing enables this carbon dioxide to be eliminated without gross change in the plasma pH. The P_{CO_2} increases and the associated increase in hydrogen ions acts on the medullary respiratory centres, CO_2 diffusing freely and rapidly into the cerebrospinal fluid (unlike bicarbonate ions). At any moment the arterial P_{CO_2} concentration is a balance of its rate of production and the rate of alveolar ventilation. P_{CO_2} has a trivial effect on dissolved CO_2, which is less than 1 mmol/l.

Renal adaptations to changes in hydrogen ion concentration, bicarbonate and chloride concentrations are slower but, combined with the rapid sensitive respiratory system, enable the plasma pH to be maintained within defined limits. The extremes compatible with life are pH 6·9–7·7, and it is worth noting that this represents a sixfold difference in hydrogen ion concentration—120–20 nmol/l.

Clinical condition	pH	[H+]	Bicarbonate	P_{CO_2}
Metabolic acidosis	↓	↑	Primary ↓	Secondary ↓
Respiratory acidosis	↓	↑	Secondary ↑	Primary ↑
Metabolic alkalosis	↑	↓	Primary ↑	Secondary ↑
Respiratory alkalosis	↑	↓	Secondary ↓	Primary ↓

Primary and secondary changes in plasma bicarbonate and P_{CO_2}, with corresponding changes in plasma pH and hydrogen ion concentration in respiratory and metabolic alkalosis and acidosis.

NON-RESPIRATORY ACIDOSIS

Non-respiratory acidosis results from a primary fall in ECF bicarbonate and fall in plasma pH (rise in hydrogen ion concentration), with a secondary fall in Pa_{CO_2} resulting from increasing depth and rate of respiration.

Signs and Symptoms

The increasing hydrogen ion concentration results in hyperventilation with initially increased depth, followed by increased rate of respiration. In severe case stupor may progress to coma.

There is depressed cardiac contractility with peripheral vasodilatation, leading to hypotension and congestive cardiac failure. The threshold for induction of ventricular fibrillation is reduced. Patients complain of anorexia and nausea, and with increasing severity, vomiting starts. There is frequently hyperkalaemia, especially if renal function is not good, as potassium ions leave the cells.

Causes

1. *Increased Hydrogen Ion Concentration*

    a Excessive production of organic acids, as in diabetes mellitus.

    b Reduced excretion of hydrogen ions, as in renal damage.

    c Excessive administration of substances such as ammonium chloride.

2. Excessive Loss of Bicarbonate Base

a   Increased loss of gastrointestinal fluids.
b   Decreased formation of bicarbonate in the body, as with acetazolamide therapy.
c   Dilution acidosis—administration of excessive volumes of isotonic sodium chloride solution, with dilution of ECF bicarbonate.

Classification of Causes on Non-respiratory Acidosis

This classification is logical, but difficult to use, since many conditions with metabolic acidosis are caused by multiple factors, e.g. aspirin poisoning, with stimulation of the respiratory centre causing respiratory alkalosis, non-volatile organic acidosis, plus ketosis and lactic acidosis.

1. Metabolic Acidosis with Normal Anion Gap (approximately 12 mmol/l)

a   *Gastrointestinal tract*
   i   Prolonged intestinal drainage; intestinal fistula ⎫ loss of bicarbonate.
   ii   Severe diarrhoea ⎭
   iii   Ureterosigmoidostomy—excessive chloride reabsorption.
   iv   Hyperalimentation, high protein diet, excess cationic amino acids. Catabolism of protein releases hydrogen ions. Hydrogen ions are released if positively charged amino acids are incorporated during protein synthesis. Infusion of L-arginine hydrochloride.
   v   Ammonium chloride orally.
b   *Renal*
   i   Early renal failure. Ability to excrete hydrogen ions reduced. Retention of sulphate, phosphate and organic acid, with incomplete reabsorption by tubules of bicarbonate.
      α   Non-bacterial interstitial nephritis.
      β   Polycystic kidney disease with a combination of reduced proximal renal tubule bicarbonate reabsorption, distal tubule inability to depress the urine pH to 5·4, and reduced ammonium production (falling from the 300–400 mmol/day found in non-renal metabolic acidosis to less than 14 mmol/day).
   ii   Renal tubular acidosis—Proximal, distal tubule defects, + Type IV, renal tubular acidosis.

iii Acetazolamide therapy—induces a gross reduction in proximal renal tubule bicarbonate synthesis and reabsorption, by inhibiting carbonic anhydrase.

iv Hyperparathyroidism—proximal renal tubule reabsorption of bicarbonate is reduced. Plasma chloride levels rise above 100 mmol/l.

2. Metabolic Acidosis with Increased Anion Gap

a Starvation ketosis.

b Uraemic acidosis—retention of phosphate, sulphate and creatinine; inability to excrete hydrogen ions adequately with reduced ammonium synthesis, retention of organic acids.

c Diabetes mellitus—accumulation of β-hydroxybutyric acid with a pK of only 2·8, acetoacetate and acetone. Complicating lactic acidosis may develop.

d Lactic acidosis
   i Tissue hypoxia and shock.
   ii Liver failure.
   iii Sepsis, neoplasia, pulmonary embolism.
   iv Drugs
       Ethanol. Excessive utilization of NAD+ with hydrogen ion formation.
       Methanol. Formate produced in the body.
       Phenformin. During treatment of diabetes mellitus, lactic acidosis can develop.
       Salicylate poisoning. Organic acidosis plus lactic acidosis.
       Antifreeze poisoning. Ethylene glycol converted into oxalic acid in the body.
       Paraldehyde excess.
       Fructose and sorbitol deplete hepatic ATP stores.

3. Metabolic Acidosis with Decreased Anion Gap

Acidosis in multiple myelomatosis—presence of excess cationic protein formed by the malignant clone of cells.

4. Mixed Metabolic Acidosis

a Endogenous organic acid production, e.g. diabetes mellitus.

b Increased loss of alkali from the body, e.g. gastrointestinal fluid loss, renal loss of bicarbonate.

c Inability to excrete hydrogen ions via the renal tract in renal damage.

Mixed metabolic acidosis combination results in hyperchloraemic acidosis with an increased anion gap.

Respiratory Compensation

The respiratory centres in the medulla are stimulated by the increase in hydrogen ion concentration in the CSF, the ventilation depth and rate being increased. The P_{CO_2} in the plasma, ECF and CSF equilibrate rapidly, but equilibration of bicarbonate takes many hours, a passive steady state between plasma and CSF being attained after about 6 h, as bicarbonate can only diffuse slowly across membranes.

In the plasma there is a rapid fall in P_{aCO_2} parallel with the fall in bicarbonate, but maximum compensation may take up to 24 h.

The P_{aCO_2} falls so that P_{aCO_2} (kPa) = bicarbonate (mmol/l)/5 + 1·1 (P_{aCO_2}(mmHg) = bicarbonate (mmol/l) × 1·5 + 8).

This is also approximately 0·135–0·176 kPa (1–1·3 mmHg) fall in P_{aCO_2} per 1 mmol fall in plasma bicarbonate. The P_{aCO_2} can fall as low as 1·35 kPa (10 mmHg).

For a plasma bicarbonate of 10 mmol/l, the compensated P_{aCO_2} will fall to 3·24 kPa (24 mmHg).

Renal Compensation

Unless there is renal damage, urine ammonium excretion following renal tubular ammonia synthesis can reach 500 mmol/day in 2–4 days. Also the urine pH can fall below 5·0 unless there is renal damage. In diabetes mellitus ketoacidosis both β-hydroxybutyric acid and acetoacetic acid can act as titratable acids, buffering an acid urine. There is increased excretion of hydrogen ion following exhange of hydrogen ion for sodium in the distal renal tubules.

Treatment

1. Treat the primary cause of non-respiratory acidosis.
2. Bicarbonate replacement may be given in an attempt to increase the ECF bicarbonate concentration. Sodium bicarbonate must be avoided in renal failure, since once it is injected the body has difficulty excreting it.

In non-renal metabolic acidosis an adult may be given 100–200 mmol of sodium bicarbonate (as 4·2 per cent solution) intravenously over a period of at least 5 min. The plasma chemistry should be checked after a futher 30 min, and this treatment can be repeated if indicated by the results. Correction of bicarbonate deficit must always be slow and

incomplete. Rapid correction is dangerous since
  a. Plasma bicarbonate 'corrected'.
$$\downarrow$$
  b. ECF bicarbonate not 'corrected'.
$$\downarrow$$
  c. CSF bicarbonate not 'corrected'. There is therefore no correction if the central respiratory drive and ventilation continue at increased depth and rate. The result is a rise in arterial/plasma pH leading to a situation of respiratory alkalosis in the blood and a persisting metabolic acidosis in the CSF and brain.

It is sensible to attempt to restore slowly a low plasma pH to above the value of 7·2, since when the plasma pH exceeds 7·2 the respiratory drive is not severe. (Various calculations have been published for the correction of bicarbonate deficit, e.g. (*a*) (0·3 × Base deficit (mmol/l) × Body weight (kg)) mmol bicarbonate, (*b*) (0·3 × (Plasma bicarbonate − 24) × Body weight (kg)) mmol bicarbonate, (*c*) (20 − observed plasma bicarbonate) × $\frac{1}{2}$ body weight (kg) mmol bicarbonate, but they all give a false sense of accuracy, and treatment should be slow, empirical, and with frequent checks of blood chemistry.)

RESPIRATORY ACIDOSIS
Respiratory acidosis results from a primary increase in ECF P_{CO_2} with a later small compensatory increase in plasma bicarbonate, the bicarbonate/carbon dioxide ratio remaining below normal, and the plasma pH falling below normal.

Causes
1 Defective ventilation
2 Defective gas diffusion in the lungs   } singly or in combination.
3 Defective perfusion in the lungs
   including
   a Pulmonary disease.
   b Airway disease.
   c Respiratory obstruction.
   d Depression of activity of the 'respiratory centre' with reduced respiratory drive.
   e Defects of respiratory nerves and/or muscles.
   f Thoracic cage disorders.
   g Inhalation of carbon dioxide-containing gases.

Signs and Symptoms

1   Fatigue, weakness and irritability.
2   Commonly headache, lethargy.
3   Depression, anxiety, confusion.
4   Somnolence progressing to delirium.
5   Abnormal EEG readings.
6   Peripheral vasodilatation, with skin warm and flushed.
7   Tremors, muscle jerks and clonic movements.
8   Heart rate increased, slowing later with increasing severity.

In pure hypercapnoea with a Pa_{CO_2} of $10.8–12.15$ kPa ($80–90$ mmHg) without hypoxia, plasma pH and CSF pH fall to the same degree. Within 1 h of the increase in Pa_{CO_2}, the bicarbonate concentration in the CSF increases and the CSF pH approaches normal values. After 3 h with a Pa_{CO_2} persisting at $10.8–12.15$ kPa ($80–90$ mmHg) the CSF pH is still below normal. Complete compensation in the CSF (and hence in the brain cells) is complete only after 4 h.

If ventilation stops, hydrogen ions accumulate at the rate of 10 mmol/min, which is 30 times the renal hydrogen ion excretion rate. Pure hypercapnoea is rare, as there is usually also hypoxia. Both hypercapnoea and hypoxia are potent cerebral vasodilators. Depression of the central nervous system is related to the CSF pH rather than to the plasma pH and in consequence there is more profound depression in severe respiratory acidosis than in metabolic acidosis. In metabolic acidosis the CSF pH is better maintained in a steady state.

Respiratory Compensation

If respiratory compensation is possible, then the ventilation rate increases with greater depth of respiration, in response to increased hydrogen ion concentration in the CSF acting on the medullary respiratory centres. Any associated hypoxia with falling Pa_{O_2} also increases respiration rate and depth, if this is possible.

With rising Pa_{CO_2}, plasma bicarbonate may rise slightly. Even if the Pa_{CO_2} has risen rapidly to $10.8–12.15$ kPa ($80–90$ mmHg) the plasma bicarbonate is only acutely increased by $+3–4$ mmol/l. If in acute respiratory acidosis the plasma bicarbonate is greater than $28–30$ mmol/l, there is also some metabolic alkalosis. Similarly, if the plasma bicarbonate is less than $25–26$ mmol/l there is also some metabolic acidosis.

In chronic respiratory acidosis, for each increase in Pa_{CO_2} of $+1.35$ kPa ($+10$ mmHg) there is an increase in plasma bicarbonate of $+4$ mmol/l, but whatever the height of Pa_{CO_2} the plasma bicarbonate rarely exceeds 45 mmol/l. The plasma pH falls below 7.35 and the urine pH is below 6.0.

Renal Compensation

The renal response to respiratory acidosis is not rapid enough to prevent changes in plasma pH and bicarbonate. Bicarbonate reabsorption and acid excretion begins by 6–12 h, reaching 90 per cent of its total potential by the third day, with stability of hypercapnoea by 3–5 days. There is renal reabsorption and retention of bicarbonate, a marked increase in urinary ammonium excretion carrying excess hydrogen ions, and a loss of chloride. A significant chloride deficit can develop in chronic cases, especially if more chloride is lost following diuretic therapy.

At first urine potassium excretion is increased, and potassium ions leave the cells to enter the ECF. The urine pH is low in the absence of renal disease.

Treatment

The cause of the respiratory acidosis should be treated if possible. When chronic respiratory acidosis is relieved, post-hypercapnoeic alkalosis develops, after the $P\text{aco}_2$ has returned to normal. Potassium chloride supplements are then required.

Correction should not be too rapid, since it takes 12–24 h for plasma bicarbonate to reach normal concentrations, following correction of hypercapnoea. If the $P\text{co}_2$ falls too rapidly to normal, and the plasma bicarbonate falls more slowly, alkalosis develops. In addition, during rapid correction the following signs and symptoms occur:

1 Hypotension.
2 Cardiac arrhythmias.
3 Sometimes tetany. Raised plasma pH with consequent low ionized plasma calcium.
4 Falling ECF $P\text{co}_2$ leading to rising ECF pH.
5 Following the rise in plasma pH there may be reduction in cerebral blood flow, with tissue hypoxia, coma and convulsions.

A patient with chronic respiratory acidosis on a ventilator, should have the $P\text{aco}_2$ maintained at a higher level by (a) adding dead space, (b) adding CO_2 to the inspired gases if necessary.

METABOLIC ALKALOSIS

Metabolic alkalosis results from a primary rise in plasma bicarbonate relative to the $P\text{aco}_2$. This can result from a depletion of hydrogen ions, or an excess of bicarbonate ions, or both. In the human body, volume homeostasis takes precedence over adjustments of acid–base equilibrium.

Signs and Symptoms

Clinical signs and symptoms are usually non-specific. There is minimal depression in depth and rate of respiration. If the degree of alkalosis is severe, reflexes are hyperreactive, with hypertonicity of muscle. This may progress to tetany, and even convulsions. Muscle weakness is present if there is severe potassium depletion. There is a risk of cardiac arrhythmia. Plasma pH is greater than 7·45, with raised plasma bicarbonate. The Pa_{CO_2} rarely exceeds 6·75 kPa (50 mmHg).

Causes

1. *Alkali Overload* (clinically rare)

The normal kidney can excrete a load of sodium bicarbonate, citrate, lactate or acetate (i.e. bicarbonate or bicarbonate precursors) rapidly. In the presence of poor renal function, such loads cause more persistent metabolic alkalosis:

  a Milk-alkali syndrome—fortunately rare. The patient with peptic ulcer ingests large doses of pain-relieving alkali plus milk. The high calcium intake may result in renal damage with calcinosis.

  b Massive bicarbonate infusion following cardiac arrest.

2. *Chloride-responsive Metabolic Alkalosis*

  a *Gastrointestinal fluid losses*

    i Gastric juice loss through vomiting or aspiration. Loss of hydrochloric acid is equal to 'gain' of bicarbonate. There is loss of sodium, potassium and hydrogen ions with greater loss of chloride (since three cations are being lost with one anion).

    ii Intestinal fluid loss.

    iii Villous adenoma of colon—large faecal loss of sodium, potassium and chloride.

    iv Congenital chloridorrhoea [R]. Excessive loss of chloride, and hydrogen ions in the stools and urine. There is also potassium deficiency and reduced EAV.

  b *Diuretic action*

    i Thiazides—weak inhibition of chloride reabsorption by loop of Henle.

    ii Frusemide, ethacrynic acid, metolazone, bumetanide and mercurial diuretics, all inhibit tubular reabsorption of chloride, with consequent loss of sodium, and hydrogen ions with chloride in the urine. Chloride is lost even when the patient is on a low salt intake. Potassium depletion develops, in the absence of replacement, and EAV falls. The fall in

EAV without proportionate fall in bicarbonate total, the bicarbonate concentration increases—*contraction alkalosis*.
iii Post-diuretic action. Chloride deficiency, potassium depletion and contraction alkalosis persist in the absence of biochemical repair.

c *Post-chronic hypercapnoea*
In patients with chronic pulmonary disease and respiratory acidosis which has persisted for more than a few days, sudden relief with fall of the raised $Paco_2$ rapidly to normal results in metabolic alkalosis. In hypercapnoea, the kidney loses chloride selectively. If there is little chloride in the diet when the $Paco_2$ suddenly falls to normal with treatment, renal acid secretion cannot be adjusted, and metabolic alkalosis persists until chloride losses are replaced.

d *Hypoparathyroidism*
There is persistent proximal renal tubular reabsorption of bicarbonate ions with excretion of hydrogen ions in the urine (the reverse occurs in primary hyperparathyroidism).

e *Glucose feeding after fasting*
A hypokalaemic metabolic acidosis develops as potassium enters the cells with glucose, during the formation of glycogen.

3. Chloride-resistant Metabolic Alkalosis

In these conditions, there is an underlying potassium depletion with chloride present in the urine (> 20 mmol/l). Plasma potassium is often < 2 mmol/l.

a Cushing's syndrome
b ACTH-producing malignancies
c Primary hyperaldosteronism

} excessive amounts of mineralocorticoid cause loss of hydrogen ions with potassium in the urine.

d Liquorice ingestion—liquorice contains an aldosterone-like substance.

e Bartter's syndrome [R]—probably a primary vascular resistance to the vasoconstrictive action of angiotensin II, which leads to raised plasma renin levels, and persistent production and release of aldosterone.

Respiratory Compensation

There is only moderate depression in depth and rate of respiration, and there is no massive rise in $Paco_2$ following the increase in plasma bicarbonate. The $Paco_2$ rarely exceeds 8·1 kPa (60 mmHg), and it is usually less than 6·75 kPa (50 mmHg). Each increase by +1 mmol of bicarbonate per litre above normal may be followed by a compensatory increase in Pa_{CO_2} of +0·07–0·14 kPa (+0·5–1·0 mmHg) up to 7·4 kPa (55 mmHg). In very severe alkalaemia central and peripheral chemoreceptors are depressed, resulting in hypoventilation, causing a rise in Pa_{CO_2}, and hence compensatory respiratory acidosis.

Renal Compensation

Renal reabsorption of sodium and bicarbonate ions in exchange for hydrogen ions does not occur in metabolic alkalosis. Potassium tends to be lost in the urine in place of sodium, leading to potassium depletion. Eventually 'paradoxical aciduria' occurs in sustained alkalosis, when hydrogen ions are excreted in the urine to save potassium. Urine bicarbonate and sodium excretion is increased, with reduced ammonium excretion. At first the urine pH is less acid than normal, but later the urine pH falls.

Treatment

The primary cause should be treated. Following gastrointestinal fluid losses, intravenous isotonic sodium chloride with potassium supplements can be given. If the patient can eat, a normal diet for a few days will normally correct the deficit in potassium and chloride. Extrapolation of results from animal experiments suggest that there is only a minimal rise in brain intracellular pH and brain lactate, with no change in brain bicarbonate.

Diuretic-induced metabolic alkalosis can be avoided in many cases by giving potassium chloride supplements with food, and the concomitant use of potassium-sparing diuretics with potassium-losing diuretics.

During recovery from severe metabolic alkalosis, the plasma bicarbonate and Pa_{CO_2} should be allowed to fall gradually together, avoiding any sudden changes in plasma (and hence CSF) pH.

If the plasma pH rises towards 7·60, this is dangerous, and active measures should be undertaken to reduce the plasma pH. Sodium chloride (isotonic) with potassium chloride supplements, with added hydrochloric acid have been given, but the solution damages veins at the site of infusion.

Lysine or arginine hydrochloride can be given orally in solution at the rate of 50–100 mmol per day. A 10 per cent solution of arginine hydrochloride contains 47·5 mmol chloride/100 ml. L-arginine hydrochloride can also be given intravenously, but this is poorly tolerated in the presence of poor renal function, and L-arginine hydrochloride may cause flushing, nausea, vomiting and headache, apart from local irritation at the injection site. Isotonic ammonium chloride has also been suggested in emergency (160 mmol/l), but toxic symptoms occur, related to the rate of infusion, including pallor, sweating, vomiting, respiratory depression and mental depression. These are particularly likely in patients with liver damage (in whom metabolic alkalosis may have developed during diuretic treatment of ascites). In patients with impaired renal function, the blood urea rises dramatically.

L-arginine hydrochloride is metabolized in the body to nitrogenous material plus free chloride ion, while ammonium chloride is metabolized to urea and chloride.

In most cases, urgent treatment of metabolic alkalosis is unnecessary, and relevant replacement of chloride and/or potassium deficit by feeding plus intravenous sodium plus potassium chloride, is sufficent.

RESPIRATORY ALKALOSIS

Respiratory alkalosis results from a primary fall in Paco$_2$ relative to plasma bicarbonate. During the period of compensation, plasma bicarbonate falls, but the bicarbonate/carbon dioxide ratio remains above normal.

Causes

1. Hyperventilation

The respiratory centre may be stimulated via the carotid and aortic bodies. If the Pao$_2$ falls acutely to 8 kPa (60 mmHg) the respiratory centres in the medulla are stimulated. If hypoxia persists, then the maximum respiratory response is reached in 4 days.

Acute hyperventilation can occur:

a   Voluntary (temporary), e.g. rapidly blowing up an air bed by mouth.

b   Psychogenic ('hysterical')

c   Excessive artificial ventilation. Each reduction of 0·135 kPa (1 mmHg) in Paco$_2$ is followed by a fall in plasma hydrogen ion of 0·75 nmol/l.

2. Less Acute, and Chronic Conditions

a   Life at high altitudes. The body adapts to chronic low Paco$_2$, e.g. 27 mmHg at 14 000 feet (4 kPa).

b   Lung disease.

c   Central nervous system disease, with stimulation of the respiratory centres.

d   Reflex stimulation from nerves in the thorax, pulmonary vessels and lung tissue.

e   Fever.

 f Drugs stimulating the respiratory centre.
   Salicylate
   Progesterone
   Epinephrine
 g Pregnancy (late stages).
 h Sudden recovery from metabolic acidosis. After a sudden increase in ECF bicarbonate, hyperventilation may persist for 12–24 h. There is delayed penetration of bicarbonate ion into the CSF, whereas carbon dioxide crosses rapidly into the CSF and, as a result, a low CSF pH (high hydrogen ion concentration) is maintained with a rising ECF pH. The hydrogen ions in the CSF stimulate the respiratory centre in the medulla.

Signs and Symptoms

1. *Acute Severe Hyperventilation*

As the plasma pH rises above 7·45, the plasma ionized calcium concentration falls, resulting in:

Dizziness
Paraesthesiae
Tetany
Myoclonus
Altered level of consciousness. Acute hypocapnoea leads to cerebral vasoconstriction and possible cerebral hypoxia. The haemoglobin–oxygen dissociation curve 'shifts to the left', reducing oxygen availability to the tissues, including the brain. The effects of any alcohol in the body are potentiated.

2. *Moderate Chronic Hyperventilation*

In some patients hyperventilation is persisted in, a 'fight-or-flight' state, with increased motor excitability and increased sensitivity to sensory stimuli, with 'paralysis by fright' in some cases. Tetany is rare, but symptoms include:

Palpitations
Precordial pain
Dizziness
'Blackouts'
Paraesthesiae, especially hands, feet and face
Dysphagia and dry cough
Heartburn
Muscle cramps
'Tension state'
Lack of concentration and sleep disturbance
Emotional sweating

Such hyperventilation may occur in passengers during aircraft flight, and also is common in opera singers.

Detection

   a. Forced overbreathing produces the symptoms complained of in 2–3 min, and the P_{CO_2} remains low for an abnormally long period afterwards.

   b. During quiet normal breathing the end-tidal P_{CO_2} shows marked variation, only minor fluctuations occurring in normal subjects.

   c. A single deep breath lowers the P_{CO_2} by 10 mmHg (1·35 kPa) and recovery takes 20–30 sec in the normal subject, much longer in a hyperventilator.

3. High Altitude

At first, at high altitude, respiration depth and rate are increased following stimulation of chemoreceptors. Alveolar oxygen increases and alveolar carbon dioxide falls, with rise in pH in both plasma and CSF, producing respiratory alkalosis.

After a few hours, following active transport of bicarbonate ions from the CSF, the CSF pH returns to normal, and respiration is again under control of central and peripheral chemoreceptors. Later, the kidneys excrete more bicarbonate. ?Mountain sickness is partially due to potassium deficiency following renal potassium loss.

Central Nervous System Pathophysiology

There is rapid migration of carbon dioxide from the neurones following the fall in arterial and CSF P_{CO_2}, resulting in increased intracellular pH, with increased neuronal activity and with electrical discharge in associated nerve fibres. Hydrogen ions cannot diffuse in and out of neurones, since they align with water molecules inside the brain cells. This occurs if the P_{CO_2} falls from 5·3 to 4·6 kPa (40 to 35 mmHg). Anaerobic glycolysis increases lactic acid production and intracellular pH falls once more, with diminution of neuronal activity, i.e. biphasic, with initial excitement followed by progressive depression, over a 2-h period.

Respiratory Compensation

In acute respiratory alkalosis following voluntary hyperventilation, e.g. blowing up an air bed by mouth as rapidly as possible, there comes a time when rapid deep respiration is no longer possible, and a period of apnoea follows. This does not occur in the other forms of respiratory alkalosis.

In acute respiratory alkalosis for each fall of $1·35$ kPa P_{aCO_2} (10 mmHg) the plasma bicarbonate concentration falls by 2 mmol/l, to a lower limit of 18 mmol/l.

In chronic respiratory alkalosis each fall of $0·135$ kPa P_{aCO_2} (1 mmHg) is followed by a fall of $0·5$ mmol/l in plasma bicarbonate, down to a lower limit of 12–15 mmol/l.

After an initial rise in brain pH, this returns to normal within 2 h in respiratory alkalosis, with an increase in lactate and organic acid concentration in the CSF.

At high altitude respiration depth and rate are increased following stimulation of chemoreceptors. Alveolar oxygen rises and alveolar carbon dioxide concentration falls, with a consequent rise in pH in both plasma and CSF. After a few hours, following active transport of bicarbonate from the CSF, the pH in the CSF returns to normal, and respiration is once again under the control of central and peripheral chemoreceptors. Later there is increased excretion of bicarbonate by the kidneys. It is possible that some part of mountain sickness is due to developing potassium depletion following loss of potassium in the urine.

Renal Compensation

Compensation takes the form of decreased net acid secretion. There is increased loss of bicarbonate ions in the urine with retention of chloride. The urine is alkaline with a high phosphate content.

In hyperventilation, the ECF bicarbonate slowly falls, until the ECF pH is normal. When hyperventilation persists, and is not due to mechanical ventilation, the medullary respiratory centre is 'reset' to produce higher minute volumes. If a low P_{aCO_2} is the result of mechanical hyperventilation, weaning the patient from the ventilator may be difficult. When the ventilator is disconnected, returning the patient to his own respiratory centre drive, high minute volumes may not be maintained. If the patient is unable to generate the necessary minute volume, the ECF pH falls below normal, the respiratory centre is stimulated, and the patient becomes distressed. Therefore the minute volume must be decreased by a small amount each day, allowing the patient's respiratory centre to 'reset' by an increase in ECF bicarbonate.

Hyperventilation can lose 3 litres of carbon dioxide in 1 h, leading to a P_{CO_2} of $2·2$ kPa (20 mmHg). After stopping hyperventilation, there is a period of hypoventilation, *but* oxygen consumption continues throughout the body all the time.

Treatment

1. Treat the cause.
2. Treatment of acute 'hysterical' hyperventilation involves rebreathing by the patient into a bag, or inhaling 5 per cent CO_2 in air.
3. If rebreathing into a bag, or breathing air $+5$ per cent carbon dioxide does not work, acetazolamide should be given. This will cause a loss of bicarbonate in the urine, and reduce the plasma bicarbonate concentration within an hour. If acetazolamide is given before ascent, mountain sickness may be prevented.

COMBINED METABOLIC AND RESPIRATORY DISORDERS

This section on combined disorders is included for completeness. In most cases a primary major condition is complicated by a secondary condition, and the diagnosis and treatment depends on the clinical history plus physical findings, aided by laboratory tests.

A. Respiratory acidosis and respiratory alkalosis is an impossible combination.

B. Acute respiratory acidosis complicating chronic respiratory acidosis presents as a sudden progressive deterioration in chronic respiratory disorder, with a dangerous fall in plasma pH (rise in hydrogen ion concentration).

C. Respiratory acidosis and metabolic acidosis is a combination with a dangerous fall in plasma pH.

D. Respiratory alkalosis and metabolic alkalosis is a combination with a dangerous rise in plasma pH (fall in plasma hydrogen ion concentration).

E. Respiratory acidosis and metabolic alkalosis

F. Respiratory alkalosis and metabolic acidosis

G. Metabolic alkalosis and metabolic acidosis

are combinations in which the plasma pH need not deviate markedly outside the normal range, but life-threatening conditions can occur.

A. Respiratory Acidosis and Respiratory Alkalosis

These cannot coexist.

B. Acute Respiratory Acidosis and Chronic Respiratory Acidosis

Cause

Sudden deterioration in pulmonary function in a patient with chronic respiratory disease, with sudden increase in Pa_{CO_2} with incomplete compensatory rise in plasma bicarbonate, and the plasma pH falling further below normal.

C. Metabolic Acidosis and Respiratory Acidosis

Findings

Increased Pa_{CO_2} with reduced plasma bicarbonate and increased plasma hydrogen ion concentration (decreased plasma pH), with no evidence of compensation.

Causes

a Metabolic acidosis developing pulmonary disease.

b Chronic pulmonary disease—developing renal acidosis; developing other forms of metabolic acidosis.

c Metabolic and respiratory acidosis developing together.
   For example:
   i Cardiopulmonary arrest followed by resuscitation: Failure of respiration and tissue perfusion results in very rapid increasing carbon dioxide retention, and accumulation of lactic acid. The very low cardiac output and poor peripheral circulation results in hypoxia and increased lactic acid production. Falling plasma pH (rising hydrogen ion concentration) blocks the beneficial actions of catecholamines, and lowers the threshold for the onset of ventricular fibrillation.

   ii Pulmonary oedema: There is initial respiratory alkalosis, but respiratory acidosis develops as fluid accumulates in the lungs. There is poor pulmonary circulation and underventilation, with increased respiratory effort. Increasing hypoxia is associated with metabolic acidosis, with lactic acidosis in severe cases.

   iii Chronic obstructive pulmonary disease with hypoxia. Respiratory acidosis plus lactic acidosis.

   iv Hypokalaemic myopathy with metabolic acidosis: When respiration is affected metabolic and respiratory acidosis coexist.

   v Hypokalaemia and phosphate depletion with metabolic acidosis occurs in diabetic ketoacidosis, and also in severe alcoholism. When muscle weakness causes respiratory impairment, then respiratory acidosis complicates metabolic acidosis.

   vi Poisoning and drug overdose: Depression of the respiratory centre results in respiratory acidosis. In severe poisoning with impaired respiration, tissue hypoxia develops with lactic acidosis. Depression of the circulation results in poor renal blood flow, and reduced renal ability to excrete hydrogen ions (renal acidosis). Metabolic acidosis due to high concentrations of organic acids occurs in:
   α Methanol poisoning.
   β Ethylene glycol poisoning.

γ Paraldehyde poisoning.
δ Toxic levels of salicylates.
   In carbon monoxide poisoning and in cyanide poisoning tissue
hypoxia is severe in spite of normal oxygen supply and normal tissue
perfusion.

Treatment

  a Treat the cause.
  b Adequate airway plus oxygen.
  c Intravenous sodium bicarbonate:
    Beware of compromised ventilation.
    Affects calcium and potassium availability.
    Beware of inducing hypernatraemia.
    Beware of inducing 'overshoot' metabolic alkalosis.
    Beware of hyperkalaemia.
    Dose: 1 mmol $NaHCO_3$ per kg body weight i.v. followed by
    plasma estimations 10 min later, and before any more bicarbonate
    is given.
  d The treatment of pulmonary oedema includes morphine, oxygen,
    diuretics and digitalis.

D. Respiratory Alkalosis and Metabolic Alkalosis

Findings

Plasma bicarbonate is abnormally high with low or normal $Paco_2$, and
a raised plasma pH.

Causes

  a. Chronic respiratory alkalosis of a moderate degree is normal in
pregnancy. This can be combined with metabolic alkalosis following
vomiting, or diuretic therapy.
  b. Patients with hepatic failure, treated with diuretics, and/or nasogastric suction with loss of gastric juice.
  c. Critically ill patients on ventilator, and treated with diuretics
and/or nasogastric suction with loss of gastric juice.

*Respiratory Disorders causing Alkalosis in Seriously Ill Patients which
Compound with Metabolic Alkalosis (see next list)*

  a. Excessive mechanical ventilation.
  b. Hypoxaemia.
  c. Sepsis.
  d. Neurological damage.
  e. Liver damage with hyperventilation.

Metabolic Disorders causing Alkalosis in Seriously Ill Patients which Compound with Respiratory Alkalosis (see list above)
 a. Vomiting.
 b. Nasogastric suction.
 c. Sodium bicarbonate infusion following cardiac arrest.
 d. Massive blood transfusion—1 unit of blood contains 17 mmol citrate, equivalent to a net gain of 17 mmol bicarbonate. One unit of packed cells contains the equivalent to a net gain of 5 mmol bicarbonate.

Pathophysiology
 A. Primary respiratory alkalosis with inadequate metabolic compensation.
 B. Primary metabolic alkalosis with inadequate respiratory compensation. Metabolic processes prevent compensation for respiratory alkalosis, and hyperventilation prevents compensation for metabolic alkalosis.

Signs and Symptoms
There is severe alkalaemia (raised pH), and this condition is a potent cause of cerebral vasoconstriction. The haemoglobin–oxygen dissociation curve 'shifts to the left' reducing effective release of oxygen to the tissues, and therefore increasing the tendency to cerebral anoxia. The cerebral effects of respiratory alkalosis and hypoxaemia are additive. If there is magnesium deficiency than cardiac arrhythmias tend to be more frequent. In alkalosis the action of parathyroid hormone on bone is impaired, and plasma calcium concentration falls. Also with alkalosis plasma potassium levels fall.

The mortality is high in patients in whom the plasma pH rises above 7·55, and when the plasma pH exceeds 7·64 the mortality rate rises to 90 per cent. This reflects the fact that the conditions causing this combined alkalosis are serious and life-threatening.

If hypoxaemia develops, then lactic acid plus hydrogen ion concentration increase, resulting in respiratory alkalosis with metabolic alkalosis plus acidosis.

Treatment
Treatment of the primary cause.

E. Respiratory Acidosis and Metabolic Alkalosis
Findings
  a. Normal plasma pH with a very abnormal HCO_3^- (high). The P_{CO_2} is higher than expected for compensation (in metabolic alkalosis).
  b. The plasma HCO_3^- is too high for the observed P_{CO_2} (in respiratory acidosis). Metabolic alkalosis makes severe respiratory acidosis worse.

Causes
  a. Chronic obstructive pulmonary disease develops respiratory acidosis. Treatment with salt restriction, diuretics plus steroids causes metabolic alkalosis. Renal bicarbonate production is increased with increased bicarbonate reabsorption. The raised plasma pH reduces the respiratory drive from the respiratory centres which in turn increases the respiratory acidosis.
  b. Metabolic alkalosis develops potassium depletion with muscle weakness. If the respiratory muscles become excessively weak, then ventilation is reduced, and respiratory acidosis is superimposed.
  c. Ventilatory failure with oedema overtreated with diuretics may develop sodium with or without chloride depletion, plus intracellular acidosis, and metabolic alkalosis. This situation is made worse by vomiting.

Treatment
  a. Treat respiratory acidosis if possible.
  b. Treat primary metabolic alkalosis with fluids, chloride and potassium replacement.

F. Metabolic Acidosis and Respiratory Alkalosis
Respiratory alkalosis with HCO_3^-, which is lower than predicted from the P_{CO_2}, suggests complicating independent metabolic acidosis. pH normal or slightly deviated.

Causes
1 Salicylate poisoning. There is respiratory alkalosis initially, due to salicylate stimulating the respiratory centres increasing 'drive'. Later there is lactic acidosis. Treat with alkaline diuresis plus acetazolamide.

2 Liver disease
   a Ammonia and other biogenic amines are thought to stimulate the respiratory centres. Progesterone which is not catabolized rapidly in liver disease also stimulates respiratory centres.
   b Hypoxaemia may develop
       i   Respiratory embarrassment by massive ascites.
       ii   Development of abnormal pulmonary vascular shunt.
       iii Ventilation-perfusion mismatching.
   c Renal tubular acidosis
       i   Alcoholic cirrhosis.
       ii   Primary biliary cirrhosis.
       iii Wilson's hepatolenticular degeneration with enhanced proximal tubular reabsorption of sodium and increased lactic acid.
3 Critically ill patients
   a Hypoxaemia
   b Cardiovascular disease
   c Fever
   d Liver disease   association of hypoxaemia
   e Sepsis   with lactic acidosis.
   f CNS disease
   g Drugs
   h Mechanical ventilator
4 Pulmonary oedema.
5 Lactic acidosis—tendency to hyperventilation—hydrogen ion action on the respiratory centres.
6 Burns cases
   a Sulfamylon used as a surface dressing of burns acts as a carbonic anhydrase inhibitor on absorption from the damaged skin, causing hyperventilation.
   b Severe burns cases often hyperventilate.
7 Pulmonary–renal syndromes
   a Goodpasture's syndrome.
   b Wegener's granulomatosis.
   c Systemic lupus erythematosus.
   d Polyarteritis nodosa.
   e Right-sided endocarditis.
   f Tuberculosis.
   g Glomerulonephritis + pulmonary oedema.
   h Renal tubular acidosis.
   i Hyperchloraemic acidoses of interstitial nephropathy + uraemic acidosis.
   Plus pulmonary involvement with respiratory acidosis or respiratory alkalosis.
8 Renal failure + congestive cardiac failure + pulmonary congestion.

9   Uraemic patient on ventilator, or overbreathing due to high blood ammonia and other amines.

G. Metabolic Acidosis and Metabolic Alkalosis
Findings

Variable results of bicarbonate, $Paco_2$ with plasma pH near normal.

Causes

1   Lactic acidosis plus vomiting. Prolonged vomiting or nasogastric aspiration leads to metabolic alkalosis. Reduced tissue perfusion if the patient is seriously ill leads to metabolic acidosis. There is a marked increase in the anion gap without appropriate compensating reduction in plasma bicarbonate.
2   Diabetic ketosis with severe vomiting.
3   Chronic renal failure with severe diarrhoea, developing vomiting.
4   Anuric patient treated without therapeutic replacement of gastric aspiration losses.
    Theoretically, this combination of disorders could be further complicated by:
    a   Respiratory acidosis.
    b   Respiratory alkalosis.

4 Kidney Structure and Function; Diuretics

     Rapid adjustments to Pa_{CO_2} and plasma hydrogen ion concentration can occur following variations in rate and depth of respiration, helping to maintain both the Pa_{CO_2} and plasma hydrogen ion concentration within a relatively small normal range.

By way of contrast, the kidney responds more slowly to deviation from the normal, with slower and longer lasting adjustments, and also a slower return to normal.

In this section the functions of the kidney are described, after a description of the structure of the nephron and its detailed blood supply. The blood supply is fundamental to the activity of the nephron with rapid diffusion of solute and water across cell boundaries in the tubular bundles. Kidney function depends on diffusion rates of individual substances at various sites in the nephron (*Fig. 5*).

Following the description of renal structure and function, the modes of action and rates of response to various diuretics are described, since diuretic therapy is universal.

KIDNEY
Structure and function
Renal blood supply
 Arterial supply
 Venous drainage
 Individual portions of nephron
  Proximal convoluted tubule
  Loop of Henle
  Distal tubule
  Collecting ducts
 Vasa recta
Glomerulus structure
Glomerular filtration
Proximal renal tubule
Loop of Henle
Distal tubule

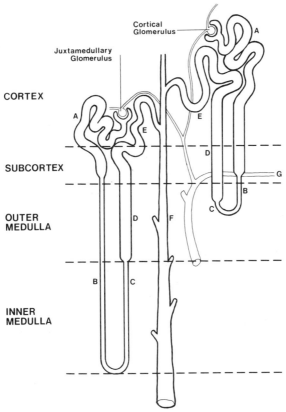

Fig. 5. Cortical glomerulus and juxtamedullary glomerulus. A, Proximal tubule.
B, Descending loop of Henle. C, Thin segment of ascending loop of Henle. D,
Thick segment of ascending loop of Henle. E, Distal convoluted tubule. F,
Collecting duct. G, Arcuate artery.

Collecting ducts
Formation of concentrated urine

Basic Structure and Function

Each kidney consists of 1–1·5 million nephrons with their blood supply.
Each nephron consists of a glomerulus, proximal tubule, loop of Henle,
distal tubule and collecting duct, and is 45–65 (average 50) mm long,
giving a very large area for absorption, excretion and exchange of water
and solute—approximately 12 sq m, which is about equal to the
corresponding renal capillary surface area. The nephrons are in
mushroom-shaped bundles, and 90 per cent lie in the renal cortex,

having short loops of Henle—the so-called 'salt wasters', while 10–14 per cent of the nephrons are juxtamedullary nephrons, with long loops of Henle reaching deep into the renal medulla—the so-called 'salt-retaining nephrons'. Tubular transit time is 2–3 min. The renal cortex contains mainly glomeruli with proximal and distal convoluted tubules, the outer medulla contains descending and thick ascending loops of Henle plus collecting ducts, and the inner medulla contains thin portions of loops of Henle and collecting ducts. There is a thick fibrous network at the corticomedullary junction, to which the renal pelvis is attached.

Kidney functions include:

a. 'Secretion' of extracellular vascular fluid, and hence ECF, with the incidental production of urine containing waste solutes plus excess water.

b. Ammonia production in association with elimination of excess hydrogen ions, in the urine.

c. Gluconeogenesis.

d. Disposal of lactate.

e. Hydroxylation of vitamin D.

f. Production of erythropoietin.

Renal Blood Supply

Arterial Supply

The total blood flow through the kidneys is about 25 per cent of the cardiac output (1200 ml/min), with 90 per cent flowing through the renal cortex and 10 per cent flowing through the medulla, a very large blood flow for organs weighing 3–4 per cent of the body weight. The blood flow can be variably distributed between renal cortex and medulla by selective vasoconstriction, and kidney activity can be measured by the renal oxygen consumption—8 per cent of the total—varying with the glomerular filtration rate and the renal blood flow.

The aortic and renal artery blood pressure ranges from 80 to 180 mmHg. Intrinsic renal control results in a constant arteriolar pressure to maintain a steady GFR. Twenty per cent of the renal blood flow is filtered. The medullary blood flow is slow, but if the flow rate increases (as in pyrexia), there is loss of the medullary osmotic gradient, with inability to produce concentrated urine, large volumes of isotonic or dilute urine being produced.

Each renal artery divides into five segmental branches, which break up into the arcuate arteries lying at the corticomedullary junction, with only capillary connections. After travelling for a varying distance, the arcuate arteries turn into the cortical tissue of the columns or the pyramidal cortex to form interlobular arteries running at right angles to the arcuate arteries. Further interlobular arteries arise from their outer convex side. The arcuate arteries are virtually end-arteries. Each nephron has its own separate blood supply, the capillary network of each kidney containing 30–40 ml of blood. The glomerular afferent arterioles arise from the interlobular arteries, which lie more or less parallel to one another, direct from the arcuate arteries themselves. The more proximal of the afferent branches arise at a recurrent angle, so that their course is directed towards the arcuate arteries. These demarcate the cortex from the medulla and supply the juxtamedullary glomeruli, the more distal of the afferent branches reach the surface of the kidney. A number of the juxtamedullary aglomerular branches run into the medulla, the arteria recta vera, which are the result of glomerular degenerations, the afferent and efferent arterioles becoming continuous. In man all glomeruli are completely developed by 12 years of age, the glomeruli in the pelvic region of the fetal and neonatal kidney disappear before adult life. Some aglomerular branches from the arcuate and interlobular arteries are found in old age and in hypertension. Each glomerulus is therefore receiving an afferent arteriole direct from a relatively large artery, the variations in arterial pressure of the large arteries (systolic–diastolic) are evened out by intrarenal mechanisms, so that the glomerulus receives a fairly constant arteriolar pressure. The right angles of the arterial branching have a significance in disease, with eddy current effects, arteriosclerosis, intravascular clotting syndromes, and immune complex deposition, affecting the junctional regions of the vessels.

The efferent arterioles from the cortical glomeruli are fine and short, and break up into the capillary plexus lying between the interlobular vessels. The efferent arterioles from the juxtamedullary glomeruli are relatively long and wide. After giving off a number of fine capillary branches to adjacent plexuses, they then divide into 12–25 descending vasa recta which enter the medulla, following the course of the loops of Henle. Many of the glomeruli giving rise to vasa recta are in the middle zone of the cortex, and therefore have a long course before breaking into vasa recta.

Venous Drainage

The capillary plexus lies around the loop of Henle in the medulla and ascending vasa recta arise from these plexuses, draining into the arcuate veins back towards the cortex. The arcuate and interlobular arteries are accompanied by single veins. The interlobular veins end in arcuate veins, and receive the wider capillaries draining the cortical capillary plexus.

Blood Supply of Individual Portions of the Nephron
Proximal Convoluted Tubule

In the subcapsular cortex the proximal and distal tubules of a nephron are usually supplied by capillary branches arising from the efferent arteriole of its glomerulus, i.e. receiving postglomerular blood from which filtrate has been removed. For the first part of the proximal tubule, the convolutions lie on the side of the glomerulus away from the interlobular vessels, where the capillaries form a freely communicating close-knit plexus. For the second part, or the more distal convolutions around the interlobular vessels, the tubule is surrounded by the terminations of the cortical capillary plexus which drains by 'coarse' or distensible capillaries into the interlobular veins. The pars recta of the terminal part of the proximal tubule is surrounded by a close-knit plexus of fine capillaries.

Loop of Henle

In the middle and inner cortex the convoluted tubule and loop of Henle are supplied by efferents from other glomeruli. Each nephron receives blood from many glomeruli, each efferent supplying a short segment. The loops of Henle which run beside the vascular bundles are part of long-loop juxtamedullary nephrons. The thick ascending loops of Henle which travel beside the vascular bundles accompany an afferent arteriole to the corresponding juxtamedullary glomerulus.

The medullary rays consist of less closely packed capillaries than in the cortex, while in the outer medulla the capillary network is most closely knit. Here numerous capillaries surround the thin descending and thick ascending limbs of the nephron. In this zone the upper parts of the long loops of Henle lie adjacent to the bundles of the vasa recta. The ascending and descending vasa recta, collecting ducts, and ascending and descending loops of Henle run together in vascular bundles. The blood flows in countercurrent to the tubular luminal fluid, to the tips of the loops of Henle and back.

The thin descending and ascending limbs that pass into the inner medulla are surrounded by a much sparser capillary plexus. The thick ascending limb passes back to its glomerulus and comes to lie between the arterioles. In this part of its course, it is surrounded by 'cortical' capillaries.

Distal Tubules

The distal tubules are intimately associated with the proximal convoluted tubules and vessels, as they are arranged in bundles of blood vessels and tubules.

Collecting Ducts

They are intimately arranged with the ascending and descending loops of Henle and are in intimate contact with the vasa recta.

Vasa Recta

The descending vasa recta carry postglomerular blood with relatively concentrated plasma proteins to the medulla. The wide distensible ascending vasa recta are important channels through which water reabsorbed from the collecting ducts is returned to the vascular system. The large number of descending vasa recta and the slightly greater number of ascending vasa recta offer a large area for countercurrent exchange in the vascular bundles. Water may be transferred from descending to ascending limbs of vasa recta by hydrostatic pressure difference. After a short course the initial branches of the juxtamedullary efferent arterioles branch into a series of descending vasa recta and a number of thin-walled veins. In this region the ascending vasa recta, having passed through the outer medulla in a compact bundle, splay out abruptly before terminating in the arcuate and interlobular veins.

The proximal vasa recta in the deepest subcortical and superficial outer medulla resemble the efferent arterioles, but are thinner. They have relatively thick endothelial cytoplasm thrown into complicated ridges and folds. The media layer is one cell thick, and there are bundles of non-medullated nerves. In the outer medulla the descending and ascending vasa recta form compact vascular bundles. There is relatively slow flow and high pressure in the descending vasa recta compared with the distensible ascending vasa recta. Each ascending vasa recta is adjacent to a number of descending vasa recta, and vice versa. The descending vasa recta with some ascending vasa recta form the central core of each bundle, with a peripheral ring of descending loops of Henle interspersed with ascending vasa recta. Outside lie a ring of thick ascending limbs of Henle and collecting ducts. The ascending vasa recta have a very thin fenestrated endothelium and surrounding basement membrane. The blood haematocrit is higher in the deeper layers of the cortex, and relatively low in the midcortex. The haematocrit increases both peripherally and towards the juxtamedullary regions (? plasma skimming occurring in the interlobular arteries).

Glomerulus Structure

Each glomerulus consists of a tuft of capillaries invaginating the thinned-out expanded proximal end of a nephron, so that the flattened epithelium forms both parietal and visceral layers. The glomerulus plus Bowman's capsule comprises the Malpighian corpuscle. The capillaries in the glomeruli have extremely thin walls, with numerous circular fenestrations, 50–100 nm in diameter. The endothelium rests on a basement membrane continuous with the cells of Bowman's capsule and continuous with the basement membrane of the afferent and efferent arterioles. The membrane consists of a dense central zone with fibrils present, and a less dense layer on either side, in all 250–420 nm thick, in man, made up of helical glycoprotein gel, tropocollagen and lipoprotein, capable of undergoing denaturation in disease. The filtering membrane for producing the glomerular filtrate therefore consists of:

1. The epithelial lining of the glomerular capillary, with open pores.
2. The basement membrane.
3. The inner epithelial wall of the glomerular capsule.

The filtering membrane has a differential permeability to molecules, very permeable to small molecules, and impermeable to large ones.

Epithelial cells, or podocytes, are applied to the outer surface of the capillaries, which can produce deposits between the cells and the basement membrane. Mesangial cells lie in the intercapillary area in the central (or stalk) region of the capillary tuft, and these cells are thought to have phagocytic functions, removing macromolecules which have not passed through the filter.

The number of glomeruli in the kidney falls in normal subjects during childhood, adolescence and in adult life. The maximum glomerular size is reached by the fourth decade. Cortical glomeruli are slightly smaller than the juxtamedullary glomeruli, with shorter afferent arterioles. In the juxtamedullary glomeruli, the afferent and efferent arterioles are continuous with glomerular capillary branches (unlike in the cortical glomeruli). The juxtamedullary glomeruli are larger than the cortical glomeruli, with longer proximal tubules, and with much longer loops of Henle, with a thin descending and ascending loop, and they have a much higher filtration rate than the glomeruli nearer the kidney surface.

Glomerular Filtration

The glomeruli act as ultrafilters producing an almost protein-free plasma filtrate. Twenty per cent of the renal blood flow is filtered, and filtration depends on the difference between the blood pressure in the glomerular capillaries and the opposing pressure exerted by the colloid osmotic pressure of the plasma proteins plus the tension in Bowman's capsule $(65 - (15 + 25))$ mmHg = approximately 25 mmHg, plus capillary permeability.

Glomerular Filtration Rate (GFR)

The GFR is determined by the balance of pressures acting across the capillary walls in the glomerulus, the plasma flow rate through the glomerulus, and the permeability and the total surface area of the filtering capillaries.

The normal GFR = 125 ml per 1·73 sq m body surface area per minute.
= 180 litres per day, of which 99 per cent is reabsorbed.
= 14 mmol solute per minute, of which 13·86 mmol are reabsorbed per minute.

a   Increased GFR

   i   Increased ECF volume.

   ii   Homozygote HbSS disease.
(Low plasma protein concentration does not cause an increase in GFR.)

b   Decreased GFR

   i   Diminished effective renal plasma flow, due to:
Reduced cardiac output.
Low blood pressure.
Renal vascular disease.
Vasoconstriction of glomerular arterioles.

   ii   Glomerular damage.

   iii   Increased capsular pressure.

   iv   Decreased functioning renal mass.

The GFR gradually falls in normal subjects with increasing age.

Proximal Renal Tubule

The proximal tubules lie mostly in the renal cortex, and the proximal tubules in the superficial cortex are half as long as those of the deeper nephrons. The proximal renal tubule has a brush border which increases the luminal surface some forty-fold. The membrane is highly permeable to urea. In both the pars convoluta and the pars recta the luminal fluid is isotonic with plasma, seven-eighths of the GFR water being reabsorbed, while one-eighth of the filtered water remains in the lumen during maximum water diuresis. With the reabsorption of salt and water, the luminal urea concentration rises, and urea diffuses rapidly into the peritubular interstitium and back into the plasma in the neighbouring capillaries. By contrast, urea is actively secreted into the luminal fluid in the straight portion of the proximal tubule.

The sodium/potassium exchange pump on the non-luminal aspects of the tubular cells, pump sodium out of the lining cells into the intercellular spaces. Sodium equilibrates with the intraluminal fluid across the 'leaky' tight junctions of the intercellular spaces, drawing water with the sodium ions out of the lumen, and entering the interstitial tissues. Electrical neutrality is maintained by active bicarbonate transfer with sodium transfer, and with passive chloride transfer. Bicarbonate, glucose and amino acids are reabsorbed in the convoluted portion.

In the proximal convoluted tubule 50–75 per cent of filtered sodium is reabsorbed, with water and urea, and 50 per cent of filtered potassium is also reabsorbed. Frusemide, ethacrynic acid, acetazolamide and thiazides are all secreted into the lumen of the pars recta. In the pars recta, some urea returns to the lumen, potassium may be absorbed or secreted, while active sodium reabsorption occurs. There is also passive reabsorption of sodium and chloride, with the development of a high luminal chloride concentration following active bicarbonate reabsorption higher up the proximal tubule. Eighty-five per cent of the filtered bicarbonate is normally reabsorbed in the proximal tubule during exchange of hydrogen ions for sodium ions. Bicarbonate generated in the proximal tubule cells releases hydrogen ions and bicarbonate ions into the tubular lumen. Phosphate and sulphate ions buffer free hydrogen ions, following sodium reabsorption with the generated bicarbonate ions. Normally 97–98 per cent of hydrogen ions excreted are consumed by luminal bicarbonate generated by carbonic anhydrase in the proximal tubular cells, and 2–3 per cent of the excreted hydrogen ions are excreted as titratable acid. Ammonium excretion governs the final urine hydrogen ion concentration.

The normal renal threshold for bicarbonate = 21–23 mmol/l in infants; 24–26 mmol/l in adults. If the luminal bicarbonate concentration exceeds this threshold, bicarbonate is lost in the urine. If luminal bicarbonate concentration is below this threshold, there is complete reabsorption of filtered bicarbonate with new generation of bicarbonate in the renal tubular cells, with an increase in urine hydrogen ion concentration (falling pH), increasing titratable acid, and increasing ammonia production and ammonium excretion.

Two-thirds of the GFR is reabsorbed in the proximal tubule without change in either the osmolality of the luminal fluid or in the sodium concentration of the unabsorbed fluid. As most of the filtered bicarbonate is reabsorbed, the chloride concentration in the luminal fluid increases progressively. Most of the filtered glucose and amino acids are reabsorbed, coupled with active sodium reabsorption.

Loop of Henle
Descending Loop
There is progressive increase in luminal fluid osmolality towards the

tip, with increasing solute addition (sodium ions). Fluid also enters isotonic to the interstitium.

Thick Descending Loop

The thick descending loop is permeable to water and impermeable to sodium and potassium. Hence water leaves the luminal fluid, the fluid becomes hypertonic, reaching maximum osmolality of 1200 mosmol/kg at the tip, when urine concentration is maximal. The loop is permeable to urea, which enters the luminal fluid from the interstitium. There is still debate on whether (1) potassium is secreted into the luminal fluid depending on the gradient from the medullary interstitium, or (2) the descending loop is highly impermeable to potassium ions.

Thin Descending Loop

The thin descending loop has a low permeability to sodium ions, and a moderately high permeability to urea and water, with abstraction of water and addition of urea to the fluid in the lumen, until the tip is reached. The surrounding medullary interstitium is hypertonic, unless there is marked water diuresis.

Ascending Loop

Thin Ascending Loop

There is low sodium and water permeability with ? active sodium chloride transport. Passive sodium reabsorption occurs because of the steep urea gradient between the medullary interstitium and the tubular luminal fluid.

The juxtamedullary nephrons have a long thin ascending loop of Henle. Following saline loading, with expansion of the ECF, there is decreased hypertonicity of the medullary interstitium. (The superficial nephrons mainly have a thick ascending limb only.)

Thick Ascending Loop

This segment is also known as the 'diluting segment'. In medullary thick limbs the luminal fluid changes from hypertonic to isotonic by the time the distal convoluted tubule is reached. In cortical thick limbs, the isotonic luminal fluid is hypotonic by the time the distal convoluted tubule is reached. The concentration of sodium chloride falls progressively, as there is active chloride reabsorption with passive sodium reabsorption at the same time. The thick limb is highly impermeable to water, and a high salt concentration develops in the outer medullary interstitium. The luminal fluid leaving the thick limb has a low salt (sodium chloride) concentration, independent of diet or the state of body hydration. This limb is also impermeable to urea.

Distal Tubule

The distal convoluted tubule begins near the corticomedullary junction. The fluid in the lumen is hypotonic or isotonic, depending on whether the loop of Henle came from deep in the medulla or less deeply. The fluid rapidly becomes isotonic. The distal tubule can variably reabsorb up to 10–15 per cent of the filtrate. Sodium reabsorption is active, and permeability for sodium, potassium and hydrogen ions is variable. In the absence of ADH the tubule is impermeable to urea and water, while during antidiuresis under the action of ADH water reabsorption is enhanced and sodium reabsorption is active. The distal tubule is closely related to the afferent arteriole of its glomerulus and also the juxtaglomerular apparatus. The maximum hydrogen ion gradient (lumen fluid : plasma) which can be maintained by the tubular cells is 1000 : 1, the urine pH falling to its lowest value of 4·4. The hydrogen ion in the distal tubule:

a 'reclaims' sodium bicarbonate

b is excreted as titratable acid

c reacts with ammonia (which diffuses freely across cell membranes) to form ammonium in the tubular lumen (which is 'trapped' there in the urine)

d (trivial amounts of free hydrogen ions).

In the early portion of the distal tubule potassium ions are pumped into the tubular cells from the interstitium and also from the lumen. In addition, potassium ions diffuse passively into the lumen according to the cell : lumen gradient. The volume of tubular fluid entering the distal tubule determines the final volume of dilute urine which can be excreted.

In the presence of ADH water permeability in the later portion of the distal tubule is greatly increased and the tubular fluid osmolality equals the plasma osmolality. Sodium continues to be absorbed actively with passive reabsorption of chloride. In the absence of ADH the distal tubule is impermeable to water, and hypotonic urine is formed with continued active salt reabsorption along the distal tubule.

Factors Involved in Distal Tubule Reabsorption

Prostaglandins (counteracting ADH).

Aldosterone enhancing sodium reabsorption at the expense of potassium excretion.

Glucocorticoids.

Angiotensin II.

Thyroid hormone.
Catecholamines.
('Natriuretic factor'—if it exists!)

Collecting Ducts

Under the action of ADH the collecting ducts become permeable to water, and water is reabsorbed, with increasing concentration of luminal fluid. Both active reabsorption and secretion of potassium can occur. Aldosterone increases sodium reabsorption with increased potassium secretion.

Cortical and antemedullary collecting ducts are impermeable to urea and water, but sodium reabsorption takes place. After a saline load there is inhibition of sodium reabsorption in the inner cortical nephrons. A concentration gradient for sodium is mineralocorticoid-dependent (e.g. salt wasting in Addison's disease and inability to excrete a water load rapidly, restored by mineralocorticoid).

The papillary collecting ducts are permeable to urea, and urea leaves the luminal fluid in the medulla. Active sodium reabsorption also takes place, depressed by increase in ECF volume.

In the terminal segments of the nephron, the highly branched papillary collecting ducts, there is continued electrolyte transfer across the cell membrane, and high permeability to water in the presence of ADH (and vice versa).

Formation of Concentrated Urine

The formation of a concentrated urine is the consequence of osmotic equilibration between the luminal fluid in the collecting ducts and the hypertonic medullary interstitial fluid. At any level in the medulla, blood in the ascending vasa recta has a higher osmolality than blood in the corresponding descending vasa recta.

Permeability to urea in the collecting ducts and in the ascending thin loops of Henle allows diffusion of urea from the collecting duct lumen into the interstitium, and hence into the lumen of the thin loop of Henle, with diffusion of water out of the lumen of the descending thin loop of Henle, drawn out by the high osmolality of the interstitial fluid.

The quantity of urea in the distal tubule is greater than the quantity of urea in the proximal tubule, maintaining high medullary interstitium osmolality, to withdraw water from the descending loop of Henle and the collecting duct. Blood in the vasa recta equilibrates with the medullary interstitium, and urea enters the vasa recta. Net reabsorption of urea beyond the proximal tubule is very small, but the osmotic pressure of the medullary interstitium maintained by salt and urea reaches more than 1200 mosmol/kg (50 per cent due to urea + 50 per cent due to sodium chloride).

DIURETICS
Osmotic diuretics
  Water
  Mannitol
  Urea
  Isosorbide
  Glucose
Acetazolamide (carbonic anhydrase inhibitor)
Frusemide
Bumetanide
Ethacrynic acid
Mercurial diuretics
Thiazides
  Chlorothiazide
  Chlorthalidone
  Metolazone and quinethazone
Xanthine derivatives
Potassium-sparing diuretics
  Triamterene
  Amiloride
  Spironolactone
Complications of diuretic
  therapy

Osmotic Diuretics

Urine osmolality approaches isotonicity with plasma. Maximum dilution of urine is impossible during the action of osmotic diuretics.

Water

When the plasma osmolality falls by more than 2 per cent, following absorption of water from the gastrointestinal tract, secretion of ADH is suppressed. The rate of renal solute excretion is not increased. Water passes from the collecting ducts into the medullary interstitium until the osmolality is equal to that of the plasma. Urine osmolality falls to as low as 40 mosmol/l (sp. gr. 1·001).

Mannitol

Mannitol, with a molecular weight of 182 daltons, is freely filtered by the glomeruli and is not reabsorbed by the renal tubules. After an infusion of 100 g mannitol as a 20 per cent aqueous solution, the ECF volume is increased, and the increase in plasma osmolality due to this amount of mannitol in an adult is only about 13 mosmol/kg. The urine volume is increased almost immediately, with normal renal function, reaching 8–10 ml per minute in hydropenics. The urine sodium concentration averages 60 mmol/l (50–70 mmol/l), and the urinary sodium excretion rate is 0·3–0·5 mmol/min.

The action of mannitol consists of inhibition of sodium and water reabsorption in the proximal renal tubule (gradient-induced inhibition), and a similar inhibition of sodium and water reabsorption in the loop of Henle (only 8 per cent of water reabsorbed, as compared with 50 per cent water reabsorption in normal untreated hydropenics). Normally in the loop of Henle 10 per cent of filtered water and 15 per cent of filtered sodium are reabsorbed. The sodium concentration falls progressively in the proximal tubule, and the luminal fluid entering the descending loop of Henle is a larger volume with relatively more water than sodium. With larger doses of mannitol, 20–30 per cent of filtered water and 10–15 per cent of filtered sodium are excreted during maximal diuresis.

Immediately after mannitol infusion the fluid in the renal cortex is hypertonic relative to the medulla, with increasing medullary blood flow and inhibition of reabsorption of urea from the collecting ducts. Osmolality of the medulla falls towards isotonicity as water passes from the collecting ducts to the interstitium. Peak urine sodium concentration can reach up to 90 mmol/l, potassium concentration reaching up to 15 mmol/l and chloride concentration reaching 110 mmol/l.

Mannitol is administered:
1 Alone
   a As a diuretic.
   b To help in the excretion of poisons which are eliminated in the urine.
   c ? to prevent renal tubular necrosis immediately following an incompatible blood transfusion.

2 With a 'loop' diuretic
3 With a potassium-sparing diuretic
4 With a thiazide diuretic

in the treatment of resistant oedema due to: (*a*) Congestive cardiac failure; (*b*) Cirrhosis with ascites; (*c*) Nephrotic syndrome.

Urea

Urea, which can diffuse across cell membranes, increases tonicity without increasing osmolality markedly, unless its concentration in the ECF is rapidly increased. When a large amount of urea has to be excreted, it produces a diuresis, reaching an excretion rate of

60 mmol/h:
1. Following high-protein tube feeding (e.g. 500 mmol/day).
2. During the early recovery phase following acute renal tubular necrosis.
3. Following oral urea treatment of SIADH—30 g urea given orally every 24 h. There is a reciprocal relationship between renal sodium excretion and renal urea excretion.
4. Intravenous infusion of urea solution has been used in the past to relieve cerebral oedema.

Isosorbide

Isosorbide is an alternative to mannitol which can be given orally. It is useful in the following conditions:
1. The reduction of raised intracranial pressure, and relief of cerebral oedema.
2. The reduction of intraocular pressure.
3. To assist diuresis in the treatment of resistant ascites in liver disease.

Glucose

Glucose in high concentration in the blood interferes with salt reabsorption, in the proximal tubule, since the normal mechanism for reabsorption of glucose in the proximal tubule is swamped by the very high concentration of glucose in the glomerular filtrate. This occurs:
1. Iatrogenic.
2. Hyperglycaemia in diabetes mellitus.

Acetazolamide

Acetazolamide is given in divided doses at a rate of 250–1000 mg per day. It acts by inhibiting the action of carbonic anhydrase, reducing hydrogen ion availability in the renal tubular lumen, and resulting in inhibition of reabsorption of sodium bicarbonate in the proximal renal tubule. This, in turn, results in an increased delivery of sodium chloride to the ascending loop of Henle. Like some other diuretics it is secreted into the lumen of the pars recta of the proximal renal tubule. The maximum rate of diuresis achieved with acetazolamide is up to 5 per cent of the filtered glomerular load. Peak urine sodium concentration reaches 70 mmol/l, potassium concentration of 60 mmol/l, chloride 15 mmol/l and bicarbonate concentration up to 120 mmol/l.

The action of acetazolamide is self-limiting, since it induces a state of metabolic acidosis, following the loss of bicarbonate ions with sodium.

Uses

Since it prevents the secretion of the aqueous humour, it is useful in the treatment of glaucoma. It may also be useful in the prevention of attacks of paralysis in familial hypokalaemic paralysis. Acetazolamide potentiates the action of:
  1. Thiazide diuretics.
  2. Frusemide.
  3. Ethacrynic acid.
It inhibits the action of aldosterone and also mercurial diuretics.

Frusemide

Frusemide is secreted into the lumen of the pars recta of the proximal renal tubule by the same mechanism as the renal excretion of PAH, and its action is completely inhibited by probenecid. In the plasma, before filtration by the glomeruli, it is carried bound to plasma protein. It acts by inhibiting the reabsorption of chloride (and hence sodium) in the ascending limb of the loop of Henle and in the proximal part of the distal tubule, and also acts as a vasodilator, increasing the rate of the medullary blood flow. Frusemide causes an increased loss of chloride, sodium, potassium and bicarbonate in the urine, acting on the tubular cells from the luminal fluid. It also causes calciuresis in proportion to the increase in sodium excretion. In doses of 20, 40 or 60 mg per dose, if given as an intravenous bolus, it begins to cause a diuresis in 15 min, with peak action at 30–60 min, its effects lasting up to 3 h. After oral dose, diuresis begins at 30–60 min, with peak activity at 2 h, and its effects lasting 6–8 h. The greatest effect is with the maximum dose. There is a modest increase in free water excretion at its peak, when urine sodium concentration reaches 140 mmol/l, potassium 10 mmol/l, chloride 155 mmol/l, bicarbonate only 1 mmol/l. The renal blood flow and the glomerular filtration rate are increased.

Uses

Following its injection as a bolus, its rapid action makes it useful as a potent agent in the treatment of pulmonary oedema. Its action persists in renal failure, even when the glomerular filtration rate is as low as 10 ml/min, if an increased dose is given. There is an abrupt loss in urine concentrating ability with a modest increase in osmolar clearance. There is also interference in the ability of the kidney to produce dilute urine. At its peak of activity up to 30 per cent of the filtered sodium load is excreted. It is effective in the presence of alkalosis with sustained loss of hydrogen ions (unlike mercurial diuretics).

Disadvantages

There is loss of potassium from cells including cardiac muscle cells, with the liability to develop alkalosis with hypokalaemia, plus an increased risk of digitalis poisoning. Carbohydrate tolerance is reduced (? associated with potassium depletion) and diabetics may require specific therapy adjustment. Uric acid excretion is reduced, especially if there is also azotaemia, and plasma uric acid concentration tends to rise with continued use. Ototoxicity occurs with very high plasma levels, e.g. after rapid intravenous bolus injection.

Bumetanide

Bumetanide has a similar action to frusemide, but is more potent. In addition, it causes less uric acid retention and less magnesium loss. It has a rapid action if given before meals, but diuresis is delayed if it is given after food. The peak blood bumetanide level when given after food is half that when given fasting, but the total diuretic and natriuretic effects are unchanged (similar results occur if frusemide is given after food).

Ethacrynic acid

Ethacrynic acid is secreted into the pars recta of the proximal renal tubule and is modified in the urine to form a cysteine complex which is 100 times as active as ethacrynic acid. The ethacrynic-cysteine complex acts on the ascending loop of Henle and the proximal portion of the distal renal tubule (similar action to frusemide), with inhibition of active chloride and passive sodium reabsorption. The onset of its action is within 20–30 min of administration, its effects lasting 6–8 h after the last dose (usually amounting to 50–150 mg/day).

Following administration of ethacrynic acid, there is an abrupt loss in the ability to produce a concentrated urine, with a modest increase in osmolar clearance. Peak urine sodium concentration reaches 140 mmol/l, with potassium concentration of 10 mmol/l, chloride concentration of 155 mmol/l and bicarbonate of 1 mmol/l. The renal ability to secrete dilute urine is also impaired. After intravenous injection the onset of diuresis is within 15 min. After an oral dose, the onset of diuresis is at 30–60 min, with peak activity at 2 h, and effects ceasing by 6 h. Unlike mercurial diuretics, the drug is active in the presence of alkalosis. Its action persists in renal failure.

Disadvantages

It can cause potassium depletion, and by promoting loss of potassium from cardiac muscle cells, increases the tendency to digitalis toxicity.

Carbohydrate tolerance is reduced, and diabetics may need specific therapy readjustment. Renal excretion of uric acid is impaired, especially in the presence of azotaemia, and plasma uric acid levels rise. On high dosage it causes diarrhoea, and there is also a risk of transient or permanent deafness.

If there is any extravasation locally following intravenous injection, the drug is actively inflammatory.

Mercurial Diuretics

After parenteral administration the diuretic is bound in the circulation to albumin. In the kidney the diuretic is secreted by the proximal tubular cells as cysteine and acetyl derivatives into the tubular lumen. These derivatives act on the cells of the ascending loop of Henle, inhibiting active chloride reabsorption (and also passive reabsorption of sodium). In the distal tubule potassium secretion into the lumen is inhibited, and sodium/potassium exchange is greatly reduced. After injection there is a delay in action lasting 30–60 min, and peak activity is reached by 2–4 h. The maximum effect is produced by a 2 ml intravenous bolus injection containing 80 mg mercury. The maximum urine sodium concentration reaches 150 mmol/l, with potassium 8 mmol/l, and chloride 160 mmol/l, and the urine contains no bicarbonate.

The mercurial diuretics tend to produce a hypochloraemic alkalosis, and after repeated administration a refractory state is induced. Activity can be increased by giving xanthine derivatives at the same time, and ammonium chloride supplements, by relieving the alkalosis, can restore their activity.

Uses

These diuretics are useful in congestive cardiac failure and in incipient pulmonary oedema.

Thiazides

Thiazide diuretics are secreted by organic acid transport mechanisms into the lumen of the pars recta of the proximal renal tubule. They act by interfering with the active reabsorption of sodium in the proximal convoluted tubule. A greater effect is exerted by interference with active sodium reabsorption in the proximal part of the distal convoluted tubule, where chloride is also passively reabsorbed with sodium, and in the collecting ducts. The maximum rate of activity is equivalent to 5–10 per cent of the glomerular load of filtered sodium. Since sodium reabsorption is inhibited, exchange for potassium ions is reduced, and there may be significant potassium loss, especially if aldosterone is active.

Chlorothiazide (250–2000 mg/day) and hydrochlorothiazide (25–200 mg/day) begin to act within 2 h of administration and continue to act for 6–12 h. Chlorthalidone (50–200 mg/day) begins to act within 2 h of administration, but continues to act for 48–72 h, and may cause problems with nocturia. The dose response to these drugs is on a fairly flat curve, and therefore an increase in dose has little effect. Cross-resistance between the various thiazides is almost invariable, and there is no point in changing one thiazide for another which has failed to produce diuresis. The thiazides, other than metolazone, are less effective when the glomerular filtration rate is less than 20 ml/min. Their effects are not abolished by either acidosis or alkalosis, and they do not cause severe volume depletion. At peak activity, urine sodium concentrations reach 150 mmol/l, potassium 25 mmol/l, chloride 150 mmol/l and bicarbonate 25 mmol/l.

Uses

They are useful in the control of essential hypertension, and recently an abnormally low sodium/potassium flux ratio has been found in erythrocytes in patients with essential hypertension. It is postulated that a similar abnormal flux is present in the plain muscle cells in arteriolar walls, and thiazides reduce muscle contraction and hence prevent an increase in peripheral resistance. In secondary hypertension the sodium/potassium flux ratio is normal. A daily dose of 25 mg of chlorothiazide is enough to control essential hypertension, and this does not cause excessive loss of water, sodium or potassium.

When thiazides are used in the treatment and control of oedema, ideally the patient should be weighed each day, and the dietary intake of sodium should be less than 50 mmol/day. In general, potassium loss in the urine is increased as the dietary sodium intake is increased, without excessive loss of chloride. When the sodium intake is kept low, there is also conservation of potassium, overriding aldosterone action.

In diabetes insipidus, especially in nephrogenic diabetes insipidus, there is a decrease in free water clearance by thiazides which cause sodium depletion. The urine volume is reduced by 50 per cent and there is reduction in the glomerular filtration rate with consequent proximal renal tubule water reabsorption.

Side-effects

Hypersensitivity reactions occur and skin rashes may appear. Thrombocytopenia develops in some cases, which recovers when the drug is stopped in most cases. Urine uric acid excretion is reduced, since the renal excretion of urates is interfered with, especially if azotaemia is present, and the plasma uric acid increases. Carbohydrate tolerance decreases possibly in association with potassium depletion, and diabetics may need specific therapy adjustment. There is also a chronic reduction in urine calcium excretion, with ECF volume contraction, and increased reabsorption of calcium and sodium in the proximal renal tubules. If sodium lost in the urine is replaced, the hypocalciuric effect is blunted, and after prolonged thiazide therapy there may develop mild to moderate hypercalcaemia.

Other Thiazides
a Chlorthalidone
Acts in the same way as chlorothiazide. It is slowly absorbed from the intestines and selectively fixed in the renal tissue. With a biological half-life of more than 40 h, its action is prolonged.

b Metolazone and Quinethazone
Act in the same way as chlorothiazide. After intravenous injection, peak activity occurs at 60 min, with action continuing for 3–5 h. After oral dosage, action begins after 1 h, with peak activity at 2–3 h, and activity continuing for 12–24 h.

Xanthine Derivatives
Methyl xanthines, especially theophylline, increase urine volume. After administration there is a transient increase in renal blood flow and in the glomerular filtration rate. There is inhibition of renal tubular reabsorption of sodium (similar action to thiazide diuretics), and peak urinary sodium concentration reaches 150 mmol/l, potassium 15 mmol/l, chloride 160 mmol/l and bicarbonate 1 mmol/l.

Theophylline potentiates the action of thiazide diuretics, and vice versa.

Potassium-sparing Diuretics
Indications
1. Primary mineralocorticoid excess.
2. Liver disease.
3. Nephrotic syndrome.
4. Severe congestive cardiac failure.
5. Essential hypertension.
6. Prevention or treatment of diuretic-induced hypokalaemia.

These diuretics can be given continuously with intermittent doses of proximal diuretics. Smaller doses should be given in the elderly, to avoid the risk of hyperkalaemia.

Triamterene

Triamterene acts by inhibiting reabsorption of sodium chloride in the distal tubule, preventing potassium exchange, and hence preventing passive diffusion of sodium ions from the tubular cells into the lumen. After oral dosage of 100–200 mg/day, diuresis starts 2–3 h after the dose, and maximum activity is reached by 6–8 h, activity persisting 48–72 h after the last dose. Peak urine sodium concentration reaches 130 mmol/l, potassium 5 mmol/l, chloride 120 mmol/l and bicarbonate 15 mmol/l. Unlike spironolactone, it continues to be effective after adrenalectomy. Since it prevents egress of potassium from cardiac muscle cells, it reduces the risk of digitalis toxicity.

Twenty-five mg hydrochlorothiazide + 50 mg triamterene has the same diuretic effect as 50 mg hydrochlorothiazide alone, but with some sparing of potassium.

Disadvantages

It may form the nucleus, or is deposited with calcium oxalate or uric acid in the renal tract. As renal stones develop in 1 in 1500 users, it should be avoided in patients with known renal stones, or with a stone-forming tendency. Smaller doses should be given to the elderly to avoid dangerous hyperkalaemia.

Amiloride

Amiloride acts by inhibiting distal tubular reabsorption of sodium in exchange for potassium. Action begins after 2–3 h, and its action lasts for up to 48–72 h from the last dose (usually 5–20 mg). The drug can be given daily over long periods, with intermittent proximal drugs (e.g. thiazides). Peak urine sodium concentration reaches 130 mmol/l, potassium 5 mmol/l, chloride 110 mmol/l and bicarbonate 15 mmol/l. The elderly should be given smaller doses to avoid the risk of hyperkalaemia.

Spironolactone

Spironolactone acts by antagonizing the action of aldosterone (which normally regulates up to 2 per cent of the filtered sodium load), and is ineffective after adrenalectomy. It acts by competing with aldosterone for binding sites on the distal renal tubular cells.

When given in continuous dosage at the rate of 25–600 mg/day, its diuretic action starts after 24 h, reaching maximum activity by 4–5 days. Its effects persist for 48–72 h after the last dose. There must be increased mineralocorticoid activity before it is effective, and it is useful in cases of hyperaldosteronism, as its action in exchanging sodium ions and retaining potassium and hydrogen ions is proportional to circulating aldosterone.

Uses

1. Useful in low-reninaemic hypertensives.
2. Useful in the treatment of oedema in the presence of hypokalaemia.
3. It can be given continuously with intermittent dosage of proximal diuretics, and can be used to potentiate the action of thiazides, or loop diuretics.
4. Useful in cirrhosis and nephrosis, both conditions associated with high levels of circulating aldosterone.

Disadvatages

1. Risk of hyperkalaemia in the elderly; therefore, smaller doses should be given.
2. There is a risk of hyperkalaemia in renal failure, and it therefore should not be used.
3. Gynaecomastia and impotence can be caused in males.
4. Healing of peptic ulcers with carbenoxolone may be interfered with.
5. Aspirin antagonizes natriuresis induced by spironolactone.

Complications of Diuretic Therapy

With excessive water loss, the EAV may fall and may cause severe hypotension resulting in renal tubular necrosis, cerebral ischaemia and encephalopathy.

Marked fall in the plasma volume results in reduced GFR, resulting in azotaemia.

The large volume of sodium presented to the distal renal tubules results in sodium reabsorption with loss of potassium and hydrogen ions, leading to metabolic alkalosis with hypokalaemia. Contraction alkalosis is liable to occur with 'loop' diuretics, especially ethacrynic acid.

Since the net loss of sodium and potassium is greater than the net loss of water, hyponatraemia develops with hypo- or hyperkalaemia (depending on which diuretic is used).

Thiazides may be associated with uric acid retention.

Diuretics can induce the hyperosmolar non-ketotic diabetic syndrome.

5 Clinical Conditions; Useful Solutions; Useful Formulae

CLINICAL CONDITIONS

Adrenocortical insufficiency
  Primary
  Secondary
Ascites
  Hepatic ascites
  Ascites in nephrosis
  Ascites in cardiac failure
Congestive cardiac failure
Diabetes mellitus
  Insulin action
  Insulin deficiency
  Treatment of diabetes mellitus
  Complications of diabetes
    mellitus
Body heat
Essential hypertension and
  sodium
Acute alcoholic hypoglycaemia
Hypothyroidism
Responses to injury, and energy
  requirements

General response
Highly catabolic patients
Enteral feeding
Intravenous feeding and its
  complications
Oedema
  Oedema
  Pulmonary oedema
  Brain oedema
Paracetamol poisoning
Renal failure
  Acute renal tubular necrosis
  Chronic renal failure with
    uraemia
  Renal Tubular Acidosis Type 1
  Renal Tubular Acidosis Type 2
  Renal Tubular Acidosis Type 4
Salicylate poisoning
Shock
Sick cell syndrome
Starvation

Adrenocortical Insufficiency

Primary Adrenocortical Insufficiency

In primary adrenocortical insufficiency, there is deficiency of both cortisol and aldosterone. This results in a slowly progressive reduction in cardiac stroke volume, plus contraction of the volume of the ECF with salt wasting in the urine, and the production of a hypertonic urine, inappropriate for the corresponding plasma sodium concentration. Urine potassium output is low, and in crisis, there is gross salt depletion, hypotension, increased cell potassium content, cell hypoxia and oliguria.

The patient suffers from muscle weakness, restlessness and insomnia, an inability to concentrate, and later, an abnormal EEG. Sensitivity to the actions of insulin increases, with hypoglycaemia and depletion of liver glycogen stores. Baroreceptors respond to the fall in ECF volume, and circulatory volume, by stimulating release of ADH. In the kidney, there is reduced GFR and enhanced proximal tubular reabsorption of filtrate, with reduced delivery of fluid to the diluting segments of the distal tubule. Both glucocorticoid (cortisol) and mineralocorticoid (aldosterone) are necessary for the production of a normally concentrated urine during hydropenia. It appears that cortisol enhances the hydro-osmotic effect of ADH in the tubular epithelial membranes of the distal nephron, by inhibiting prostaglandin generation, and its deficiency impairs the ability to produce dilute urine. A patient with Addison's disease is unable to excrete a water load efficiently.

The impairment in renal diluting ability with inability to excrete a water load efficiently is partially compensated for, if an adequate salt intake can be maintained, sufficient potassium being excreted to maintain potassium balance (i.e. salt craving in Addison's disease). Reduction in the medullary blood flow also decreases the kidney concentrating and diluting abilities.

Treatment

In addition to an adequate salt intake, cortisol 20 mg a.m. and 10 mg p.m. are given, controlled by estimated ideal plasma cortisol levels of:
1. One hour after the morning dose—700–1000 nmol/l.
2. One hour before the evening dose—350–400 nmol/l.
In all but mild cases, fludrocortisone 0·1–0·2 mg is given on alternate days.

Secondary Adrenocortical Insufficiency

Adrenocortical insufficiency secondary to pituitary disease results in ECF hyponatraemia due to dilution, with inability to excrete a water load normally, inability to form a maximally dilute urine, and inability to attain the maximum rate of diuresis, with consequent risk of water intoxication. The patient suffers from nausea, abdominal pain, hypotension, and later, mental disturbance. Plasma cortisol and ACTH levels are low, and there is no gross saline depletion or dehydration, as aldosterone is still formed in the adrenals. There is no pigmentation.

Treatment

Cortisol replacement is required, as in primary adrenocortical insufficiency. In addition, thyroxine replacement is usually required, with regular control serum checks of thyroid function. Serum T_4 levels should be kept at the upper limit of normal (in the absence of cardiac disease), and an abnormally raised TSH indicates insufficient thyroid replacement therapy.

Ascites

Hepatic Ascites

In portal hypertension the venous outflow from the liver is impeded, with distension of the portal circulation and increased portal pressure. There is decreased venous return to the heart, with reduced cardiac output and consequent renal conservation of sodium and water. The portal pressure rises until the venous return to the heart is restored. There is also an increased flow of lymph. At this stage patients are unable to excrete a sodium load efficiently. With the increasing portal pressure, fluid is filtered as a transudate from the splanchnic bed capillaries into the peritoneum to form ascitic fluid. There is probably altered permeability of the subperitoneal capillaries, and there is debate as to whether lymph contributes to ascitic formation in portal hypertension. A simple increase in portal pressure does not usually cause ascites, and formation of ascitic fluid may be increased when the capacity of the lymphatics to drain the excess fluid away is exceeded. In decompensated cirrhosis the EAV is reduced and renal retention of sodium and water makes the clinical state worse, in the absence of diuretic therapy.

Hyponatraemia results in aldosterone release, which is not catabolized as rapidly as normal in liver disease, and its action is therefore prolonged. Decreased EAV also results in release of ADH, with further water retention. Renal excretion of sodium and water is less than intake and, during accumulation of ascites, the urine sodium concentration is very low (in the absence of diuretic therapy).

Theories of Ascitic Fluid Formation and associated Hyponatraemia

1   *Sodium retention secondary to ascites formation*
    Loss of fluid into the peritoneal compartment and pooling of blood in the splanchnic circulation results in reduced effective extracellular fluid volume and reduced blood volume, with consequent reduction in renal perfusion, and sodium retention by the kidneys:
    a Activation of the renin–angiotensin–aldosterone system.
    b Reduced GFR with renal sodium retention (but often, the GFR is normal or increased in cirrhosis).
    Also total body exchangeable sodium content is increased by + 10–25 per cent in patients without ascites.

c   Spontaneous disappearance of ascites can occur in cirrhotics, without any change in either plasma volume or portal pressure.

2   *Sodium and water retention is the primary cause of ascites*
There is expanded overflow of ECF into the peritoneal fluid. The balance of the plasma oncotic pressure, portal pressure and hepatic lymph drainage favours fluid transudation into the peritoneal cavity, even without acute increase in total exchangeable sodium. Favouring this, it has been found that the sodium-retaining mineralocorticoid, 9α-fluorohydrocortisone induces ascitic formation in cirrhotics. Also following portacaval shunt there is reduction in portal pressure, and ascites is replaced by peripheral oedema (i.e. sodium is still being retained).

3   *Renal*
Patients forming ascites have circulating aldosterone in blood (and excretion in the urine) and sodium retention is reversed with spironolactone therapy or there appears to be increased sensitivity of renal tubule cells to aldosterone action. The presence of a natriuretic hormone (as yet not isolated) has been postulated as causing:

a   Intra-renal redistribution of renal blood flow to the juxtamedullary glomeruli, at the expense of the cortical glomeruli.

b   Sodium receptors in the portal venous system not stimulated as a result of portasystemic circulation shunts in cirrhosis.

Ascites in Nephrosis

Ascites is associated with peripheral oedema. The renal excretion of salt and water is less than intake. There is marked reduction in plasma oncotic pressure due to low plasma protein concentration (especially albumin reduction), following excessive loss in the urine. The effective arterial volume falls, and in the absence of diuretic therapy, urine sodium output falls.

Ascites in Cardiac Failure

Ascites is associated with peripheral oedema, which results from circulatory changes, including reduced EAV.

Congestive Cardiac Failure

In the early stages cardiac output at rest may be normal, but output fails to increase appropriately during exercise, with an abnormal rise in ventricular end-diastolic pressure and little change in the stroke volume. The result is a reduced effective circulatory volume, with redistribution of blood flow to vital organs and reduced blood flow to the kidneys, mediated by neurogenic reflexes. There is then appropriate release of ADH with water retention. Underperfusion of the kidneys with reduced GFR is followed by retention of sodium plus water by the proximal renal tubule. Decreased delivery of sodium and water to the loop of Henle dissipates the normal medullary concentration gradient, and reduces the power of the kidney to concentrate urine. At this stage urine sodium concentration is less than 10–15 mmol/l (in the absence of diuretic therapy) with a urine osmolality of 350–400 mosmol/l.

With deterioration, cardiac output cannot be augmented to meet the requirements of normal activity and there is increasing sodium retention. Sodium retained during the day is eliminated incompletely in the evening at rest. The body weight at this stage is increasing. The total plasma volume and the venous filling pressure both increase in an attempt to maintain an effective circulating volume, with increasing venous backpressure. Peripheral oedema develops, with increased fluid accumulating in the lungs, breathlessness and right-sided heart failure. Cardiac output is below normal at rest in the late stages of failure. There is persistent generalized peripheral vasoconstriction, with a further deviation of blood flow from the kidneys (which normally take 25 per cent of the total cardiac output) to vital organs. The glomerular filtration rate and the renal blood flow being low, there is a reduced luminal filtrate which is excessively reabsorbed, and sodium retention persists.

The retention of sodium and water, with peripheral oedema, is accompanied by the passage of urine with an increasing osmolality but with a low sodium content (in the absence of diuretic therapy). The patient is unable to excrete a water load rapidly and hyponatraemia follows when fluid intake exceeds fluid output. In patients passing dilute urine, the non-osmotic stimuli for release of ADH is overridden by osmolar suppression of ADH release by fall in plasma osmolality. Venous pressure increase with reduced effective circulating volume due to reduced cardiac output results in non-osmolar release of ADH. Venous pressure rise plus continuous loss of potassium from body muscle cells stimulates aldosterone release, with further sodium retention. The reduced GFR also results in continued sodium and water reabsorption.

Increased left atrial pressure with distension of the pulmonary capillaries and fluid transudation, causes increased respiratory effort with dyspnoea. Patients with detectable circulating ADH have been found to have raised blood urea concentrations with increased urea/creatinine ratios, which are not diuretic-induced. In patients without detectable circulating ADH, the blood urea levels are not so high, and it is worth noting that the plasma urea is a useful index of the severity of cardiac failure and its response to treatment.

It has been suggested that ADH is released in patients with

predominantly right-sided heart failure, but not released in predominantly left-sided heart failure. This begs the question of belief in the distinction between right- and left-sided heart failure. Treatment consists of bed rest, diuretics and a palatable diet with salt intake limited to 90 mmol/day (i.e. no added salt at table). Fluid restriction is ideally limited to daily fluid losses plus 500 ml per day, but this may cause severe thirst. Digitalis is used if atrial fibrillation requires control, but the use of digitalis when rhythm is normal is debated.

Diabetes Mellitus
Insulin Action
1 Inhibits the lipolysis of triglycerides from adipose tissue. Counteracts lipolysis stimulus of:
   a ACTH.
   b Cortisol.
   c Glucagon.
   d Beta-catechols.
   e Human growth hormone.
2 Fosters production of glycerophosphate, and hence re-esterification of free fatty acid (FFA).
3 Inhibits keto acid formation.
4 Promotes the utilization of keto acids by non-hepatic tissue.
5 Permits utilization of glucose through the pentose phosphate pathway, providing the NADPH necessary for fatty acid synthesis from acetyl-CoA.

Insulin Deficiency
1 Known diabetic patient misses taking insulin dose.
2 Infection increases insulin requirement in diabetic.
3 Surgery, trauma, myocardial infarction and burns all increase the insulin requirement in a diabetic.
4 Abrupt failure of insulin production, as in juvenile diabetes mellitus.
5 Abrupt failure of insulin production, occasionally in acute haemorrhagic pancreatitis with destruction of the pancreas.
6 Antagonism to insulin action:
   a Cushing's syndrome.
   b Thyrotoxicosis.
   c Phaeochromocytoma.
7 Massive overeating debauch in a latent or subclinical diabetic.
8 Chronic repeated excess insulin dosage leading to depletion of all liver glycogen.

Pathophysiology
1. Impaired utilization of glucose by all tissues except the brain.
2. Excessive production of glucose from non-carbohydrate sources.
3. Marked rise in ECF glucose concentration, and since the cell membranes are impermeable to glucose, hyperosmolality of the ECF.
4. The hyperosmolality of the ECF draws water out of cells, tending to dilute ECF sodium. Vomiting, which commonly occurs in diabetic ketoacidosis, causes loss of chloride.
5. When the hyperglycaemia exceeds the renal threshold for glucose, there is an osmotic diuresis with glycosuria. This loss of glucose can reach 278 mmol/h (50 g/h), and water is progressively lost from the ECF. An increase in plasma osmolality of $+10$ per cent represents a loss of 10 per cent total body water. There is polyuria and polydipsia (in the conscious patient).
6. There is tissue breakdown in a starvation-like state, with hyper-secretion of adrenal glucocorticoid. With rapid glycogen depletion from the liver, for each 3 g of glycogen removed from store, 1 mmol of potassium is released into the ECF. Glycogen (200–300 g) released as glucose is accompanied by 70–100 mmol of potassium into the ECF.
7. As water leaves the cells, potassium, magnesium and phosphate are also lost from the cells. (Insulin is required normally to maintain the highest optimal ICF/ECF potassium ratio.) Aldosterone secretion which follows the severe sodium depletion results in further loss of potassium in the urine. Vomiting prevents potassium-containing foods being eaten, and potassium from gastric juice is lost. There is therefore a severe potassium depletion.
8. Urinary sodium and chloride concentrations are about 50–100 mmol/l, causing severe sodium depletion, but concentrations fall to 10–25 mmol/l later, as the GFR and renal blood flow fall with dehydration and circulatory collapse, with oliguria, progressing to anuria.
9. Triglyceride lysis by lipase occurs, producing free fatty acids (FFA) (normally inhibited by insulin action).
10. The liver cells take up the liberated FFA, and form coenzyme-A derivative in the cytosol. Glucagon increases entry of FFA into the mitochondria for oxidation. Aceto-acetic acid accumulates from acetyl-CoA, some of which is slowly and non-enzymatically converted to acetone, which is poorly eliminated from the circulation.
11. Aceto-acetic acid is reduced to form β-hydroxybutyric acid. The relative concentrations of aceto-acetic acid and β-hydroxybutyric acid depend on the availability of NADH. The NADH/NAD ratio is proportional to the β-hydroxybutyric acid/aceto-acetic acid ratio and this latter ratio is normally 2 : 1. β-hydroxybutyric acid does not react with nitroprusside. If response to increased fluid intake plus insulin

results in increased tissue perfusion and oxygenation with increased availability of NAD, the negative-reacting β-hydroxybutyric acid is converted to aceto-acetic acid, and the 'test for ketones' becomes positive even though the patient is clinically improving.

12. There is rapid excretion of these ketone acids in the urine if kidney function is normal, with ketonuria without ketonaemia. The reverse occurs if there is renal failure, with ketonaemia without ketonuria.

13. The liver cannot metabolize the ketone acids it synthesizes. They are taken up by muscle, kidney cells, etc. and oxidized to carbon dioxide and water (although this is depressed in uncontrolled diabetes).

14. Progressive metabolic acidosis develops, with consumption of bicarbonate and falling plasma bicarbonate concentration (with therapy, muscle converts ketone bodies to bicarbonate). The anion gap rises as more organic acid is produced.

15. The plasma pH falls, and respiration is stimulated, resulting in the so-called 'Kussmaul respiration'—deep and slow. Maximum respiratory response to the acidosis takes 12–24 h to develop. The Pa_{CO_2} falls secondarily in compensation.

16. The urine pH falls, with increased phosphate and ammonium excretion, in an attempt to eliminate the excess hydrogen ions.

Treatment

In summary, this consists of:

1   Continuous infusion of insulin at the rate of 5–10 units per hour.
2   Correction and maintenance of sodium, chloride and potassium depletion.
   a   One litre of isotonic saline in the first hour.
   b   One litre of saline with 40 mmol of potassium in 4 h. Then assess.
   c   At least 4–5 litres of fluid during the first 24 hours.

Complicated Diabetes Mellitus

1   Metabolic keto-acidosis plus metabolic alkalosis due to:
   a   Severe vomiting.
   b   Excessive bicarbonate therapy. Since bicarbonate takes at least 6 h to equilibrate across into the CSF, the pH of the CSF can fall lethally.
2   Keto-acidosis plus respiratory alkalosis. Respiratory infection is common in diabetics, with hyperventilation.
3   Hyperosmolar non-ketotic coma: Treat as above, but do not allow the plasma glucose concentration to fall below 16 mmol/l during the first 12 hours, as there is great danger to the brain cells if

osmolality falls suddenly. Fluid deficit should be repaired with 0·45 per cent and isotonic saline alternately, with added potassium supplements, giving up to 9 litres in the first 24 hours. During treatment, the reduction of plasma glucose by 3·5 mmol/l is accompanied by a concomitant rise in plasma sodium of 1 mmol/l, e.g. reducing plasma glucose from 47 mmol/l to 12 mmol/l is associated with a rise in plasma sodium of 10 mmol/l. If the initial plasma sodium concentration was 150 mmol/l, it rises to 160 mmol/l unless treated. The water deficit in a 70-kg man rises from:

$$\frac{70}{2}\left(1 - \frac{140}{150}\right) \quad \text{to} \quad \frac{70}{2}\left(1 - \frac{140}{160}\right)$$

i.e. from approximately 2·5 litres to 7 litres.

4   Lactic acidosis
   a   Hypotension and shock, with poor tissue perfusion.
   b   Fructose therapy.
   c   Phenformin therapy.

5   Hyperlipidaemia
   In poorly-controlled insulin-dependent diabetic children, plasma sodium, potassium, chloride, bicarbonate estimations may be spuriously low, if there is marked displacement of plasma water by lipid. Failure to recognize this error has led to the administration of sodium chloride plus potassium supplements, resulting in severe true hypernatraemia associated with confusion and convulsions, with potential brain damage.
   This can be avoided by:
   a   Recognizing the thick layer of lipid on top of spun plasma.
   b   When diluted plasma is sprayed through a flame photometer for sodium and potassium estimation, the true plasma sodium and potassium concentrations can be calculated via a serum triglyceride correction factor.
   c   The lipids can be extracted in carbon tetrachloride, and sodium and potassium concentrations estimated from the aqueous phase.
   d   Plasma osmolality is not affected by lipid. Therefore there is a gross discrepancy between the measured plasma osmolality and the osmolality calculated from the photometer results.

Body Heat

In basal rate of heat production, the body produces 60–70 Kcal per hour. During intense physical work, this can increase to 1000 Kcal per hour. Body heat exchange with surroundings takes place by radiation and convection at first. Loss by conduction is negligible, except during exposure in cold water. If the heat which needs to be lost exceeds that possible by radiation and convection alone, then perspiration occurs, with evaporation and consequent heat loss.

Acclimatization to external heat resembles physical conditioning. Both exposure to external heat and hard physical work result in release of aldosterone. Similarly both heat exposure and hard work are followed by reduction in the GFR and in urine production. Exposure to heat is followed by hyperventilation with a fall in Paco$_2$ and plasma potassium concentration. Plasma phosphate also falls without any increase in urine phosphate excretion. Acclimatization results in a low normal plasma potassium level, without potassium depletion.

Essential Hypertension and Sodium

Recently much interesting work has been published relating sodium metabolism to essential hypertension.

1. In communities that consume large quantities of salt there is evidence that in essential hypertension and also in increased blood pressure associated with age, there is an increase in the circulating concentration of an inhibitor of sodium/potassium ATPase (? in genetically susceptible subjects).

2. In a proportion of patients with essential hypertension there is a change in the sodium/potassium flux across red cell membranes (and probably across other cell membranes). It has been suggested that such an abnormality in plain muscle cells in the walls of small arteries could be associated with increased vascular resistance and hypertension.

3. It is thought possible that raised intracellular sodium concentration in vascular smooth muscle cells could influence the intracellular free calcium concentration, acting as an immediate trigger of muscle contraction, resulting in vasoconstriction and increased blood pressure.

4. In essential hypertension there is reduced effective renal plasma flow through the cortical nephrons (the 'salt wasters'), the plasma flow through the juxtamedullary nephrons being maintained (the 'salt retainers'). ? Genetic fault.

5. Essential hypertension patients given a low sodium diet (50 mmol/day), with a high potassium content in diet (200 mmol/day), have a significant reduction in blood pressure rise induced by noradrenaline.

6. A proportion of patients with essential hypertension treated with thiazides require potassium supplements, or an abnormally low plasma potassium concentration develops (? related to sodium/potassium ATPase defect).

Acute Alcoholic Hypoglycaemia

After a period of fasting sufficient for liver glycogen stores to be depleted, even a moderate amount of alcohol without adequate carbohydrate intake at the same time can cause hypoglycaemia severe enough to impair function dangerously, e.g. driving after a 'short' drink just before lunch, and after a light early breakfast. This type of hypoglycaemia can develop with a blood alcohol of not more than $25\,mg/100\,ml$.

Oxidation of alcohol in the cell cytosol of the liver generates NADH at the expense of NAD^+, and the $NADH/NAD^+$ ratio rises, diminishing gluconeogenesis via oxalo-acetate.

Reactions depressed by Alcohol Catabolism

1. Fatty acid oxidation.
2. Citric acid cycle activity.
3. Gluconeogenesis.
4. Albumin synthesis.
5. Drug catabolism.
6. Folate metabolism.

Reactions enhanced by Alcohol Catabolism

1. Ketone body formation.
2. Uric acid formation.
3. Porphyrin synthesis.

Hypothyroidism

In addition to the reduction in the basal metabolic rate, reduction in T_4, T_3, and increases in TSH and serum cholesterol levels, these patients excrete a water load abnormally slowly, and may develop a syndrome resembling SIADH, possibly caused by:

1. Reduction in plasma volume with increased ISF.
2. Central effect of thyroid hormone deficiency may cause secretion of ADH, with consequent water retention.
3. Reduced cardiac output results in reduced GFR and reduced delivery of solute and water to the diluting segment of the nephron, with salt and water retention.

The creatinine clearance is normal or slightly reduced, with normal plasma potassium and bicarbonate levels. Urine sodium excretion is low, with increased urine osmolality.

Response to Injury, and Energy Requirements
General Response

Following injury, the rate of body protein breakdown is proportional to the severity of the injury or the surgical operation. Protein catabolism is increased by any infection and lasts as long as injury or complications persists.

Pain and trauma trigger release of ADH and aldosterone in the acute phase, and for the first few days after surgery, fluid conservation by the body overrides responses to tonicity changes in the body fluids. There is also release of cortisol and glucagon, with catecholamine-mediated suppression of insulin secretion and a period of resistance to the action of insulin with carbohydrate intolerance, especially after burns.

If the catabolic rate is increased, then treatment with insulin and glucose reduces the body protein catabolism.

In the chronic phase of stress due to injury, aldosterone and ADH release also occurs, with isotonic and hypotonic expansion of the ECF (the so-called 'hyponatraemia of the sick patient').

A starving patient during the postoperative period with a complicating infection may consume 5000 calories per day, and losing weight at the rate of 1 kg per day, has lost 10 per cent of his body weight after 7 days. No change in body weight or weight increase in the first few days after operation or injury indicates fluid retention. Starvation complicating the acute illness of injury has a high death rate when 25 per cent of the body weight has been lost, and feeding fails to reverse the metabolic consequences of injury. A total of 250–400 g of muscle plus 150–200 g of body fat may be catabolized daily.

In the immediate postoperative period, if facilities for accurate weighing are available, body weight losses of less than 300 g per day or gains of less than 150 g per day represent calorie loss of body tissues, whereas body weight losses exceeding 300 g per day, or gains greater than 150 g per day, represent fluid loss or gain plus calorie loss. During the first 48 hours after surgery, the fluid intake should not exceed 1 litre of isotonic saline + 1·5–2 litres of 5 per cent glucose solution per day, to include 40–60 mmol of potassium, plus fluid replacement of fluid losses (e.g. gastric aspirate). Fifty grams glucose yield 170 calories, and is protein-sparing. One hundred grams dextrose per day reduce urinary nitrogen loss from 10–15 g per day to 3 g per day. Even 3 litres of fluid per day may be excessive, especially in elderly patients, since in the immediate postoperative period there is a period of antidiuresis. Overenthusiastic 'fluid replacement' plus diuretic therapy embarked on during the first 48 hours after operation, to force a flow of urine, is one of the commonest causes of severe hyponatraemia with fluid retention in hospital practice—not SIADH (syndrome of inappropriate antidiuretic hormone release) but SOIA (syndrome of overenthusiastic iatrogenic activity). Weight loss during the first few days is acceptable, until not more than 10 per cent of the body weight has been lost. By then, the period of natural antidiuresis will have ceased, and the patient may be able to take food and drink by mouth once more.

If intensive feeding is necessary, various feeding regimes are available. Glucose at the rate of 25 g per hour, with insulin 10–20 units per hour, with the blood glucose maintained between 3 and 20 mmol/l, has been used in severe trauma and burns cases with marked potassium and nitrogen loss.

Using tube feeding or intravenous feeding it takes 3 weeks of intensive feeding to increase a low serum albumin in an injured patient with otherwise normal liver function.

It has been found that burns cases with control of their environmental temperature raise their room temperature to at least 32 °C, shivering at ordinary temperatures, and it has been suggested that such patients should be nursed at 32 °C to reduce body heat production, and reduce calorie loss.

High Hypercatabolic Patients

1. Major burns
2. Severe sepsis
3. Severe trauma   } singly or in combination.
4. Multiorgan failure
5. Acute renal failure

The body may be consuming 3000–5500 calories per day:
1. Heat production.
2. Evaporation of water from surfaces.
3. Catabolism of muscle.

The loss of heat from the body is the reason for keeping the room temperature at the patient's thermoneutral temperature (25–28 °C) after severe burns. After injury there is a short period of depressed vitality with reduced metabolic rate, lowered body temperature and reduced cardiac output. This is followed by a short phase directed by cortisol, followed by a phase directed by catecholamines and glucagon.

Hepatic glycogen can only supply about 800 Kcal and stores are exhausted in the first 12 hours after injury. Protein stores in muscle contain a potential 20000 Kcal representing up to 10–12 days' supply of energy. The fat stores can provide up to 130000 Kcal representing 20–25 days' supply of energy. The basal resting energy requirement in the absence of injury or illness is about 1800 Kcal/day, but can increase to 5500 Kcal/day in a hypercatabolic patient.

When a patient is unable to take food and drink actively, it is possible to give enteral feeds via a nasogastric tube.

1. *Enteral Feeding*

Starting gradually with not more than 25 per cent of the estimated day's requirement on the first day, and gradually building up to 100 per cent requirement of energy by the fifth day, enteral feeding can at least reduce the devastating body wasting which rapidly progresses in hypercatabolic patients. The low-residue diet supplies the necessary glucose (frequently in the form of the polymer, Caloreen), protein, oligopeptides, amino acids, electrolytes and trace elements plus vitamins. Abdominal cramps and diarrhoea are complications.

Plasma sodium, potassium, chloride, bicarbonate and urea estimations, and liver function tests should be carried out regularly. The volume and content of all fluids lost from the body should be measured, so that an accurate balance can be maintained. If a glycosuria exceeds 0·5 per cent or blood glucose exceeds 10 mmol/l, insulin should be given on a sliding scale.

2. *Intravenous Feeding*

Indications

 a Preoperatively, to correct existing nutritional deficiencies, e.g. in cases of carcinoma of the oesophagus. It is hoped to reduce the effects of the postoperative hypercatabolic phase in these wasted patients.
 b Chronic feeding.
   i   Short bowel syndrome.
   ii Crohn's disease.
   iii Ulcerative colitis.
 c Partial or complete failure of gastrointestinal function.
 d Acute hypercatabolic patients.

Such therapy via a central line should be started gradually (to prevent gross hyperglycaemia) and should be discontinued slowly (to avoid dangerous rapidly-developing severe hypoglycaemia).

The feed contains glucose (and at least 30 per cent of the calories given, should be in the form of glucose). Insulin may well be required, if there is 'insulin resistance' and hyperglycaemia.

Fat is given as Intralipid, and not more than 2 g fat/kg body weight/day should be given. It is important that the plasma is checked to see whether fat is being satisfactorily cleared from the plasma. Up to 8 per cent of the calories required can be given in this form of fat.

Pre-protein nitrogen is given in the form of L-amino acids, and glucose, fat and amino acids must be given simultaneously.

Minerals, including sodium, potassium, calcium, magnesium salts, phosphate, traces of zinc, plus vitamins, are required in a full intravenous diet. Plasma sodium, potassium, chloride, bicarbonate, urea and full blood count (with check on plasma for uncleared fat) estimations are required daily. Every 3 days, liver function tests should be performed, and 24-h urine excretion of sodium, potassium and urea are required not less than every 3 days.

Complications

Intravenous feeding is potentially dangerous:

a Infection—septicaemia via the catheter.

b Hyperosmolality.

c Rebound hypoglycaemia, which appears very rapidly if hypertonic glucose infusion is stopped quickly (e.g. drip stopped for 15 min).

d Low plasma potassium and inorganic phosphate, especially after insulin.

e Metabolic acidosis from acidic amino acids.

f Deficiency or overdose of vitamins.

g Decrease of antibody production following reticulo-endothelial trapping of fat particles, with risk of infection.

h Trapping of fat particles in the lungs with reduced Pao_2.

i Sudden reduction in metabolism of fat if Gram-negative septicaemia develops.

j Metabolic insufficiency—severe hyperglycaemia develops rapidly, as the infusion is entering the systemic circulation directly, rather than via the portal system (normally from the intestines). The peripheral tissues may be subjected to prolonged grossly abnormal hyperglycaemia.

k A hypercatabolic patient who is still able to mobilize fat stores following stress may develop ketosis plus lactic acidosis, with release of insulin. This results in inability to metabolize exogenous triglyceride, and at this time fat may not usefully be infused.

l Plasma magnesium may fall markedly.

Oedema

Accumulation of inappropriate interstitial fluid outside the plasma space, but including pleural effusion and ascites, may be local or general. Pitting oedema which is not due to a local lesion represents the accumulation of an additional 3–4 litres of fluid in the ECF.

Normally blood passes from an arteriole into a meta-arteriole into a preferential channel which loops back from itself, and from which arise two capillary branches leading to the venous side of the preferential channel, a venule, and then into a muscular venule. The calibre of the capillaries is controlled by sphincters on the arteriolar side, which open and shut rhythmically—in the open position, fluid is forced out into the ISF and in the shut position fluid flows inwards into the capillaries. The lymphatics start as small tubes, which flow together, becoming confluent to form larger lymphatics, and eventually the thoracic duct opening into the left subclavian vein, and lymphatics opening into the right subclavian vein.

Causes

1 Raised capillary pressure, due to increased venous pressure:
    Local.
    General, e.g. CCF.
    ISF accumulates when the rate of addition of fluid exceeds the rate at which the lymphatics can carry it away (raised capillary pressure plus force of gravity).
2 Raised plasma oncotic pressure:
    Low plasma albumin.
    Dilution of plasma protein by retained water.
3 Increased interstitial fluid colloid osmotic pressure.
4 Increased capillary permeability:
    a Action of toxins ⎫
    b Metabolic factors ⎬ capillary size increased.
    c Physical force ⎭
5 Altered tissue pressure—lowest where connective tissue strands least, e.g. periorbital tissues and oedema in fluid retention in acute glomerulonephritis.
6 Inhibition of precapillary sphincters:
    a Drugs.
    b Toxins.
    c Inflammation.
    d Trauma.
7 Obstruction of lymphatics.

Specific Clinical Conditions

1. *Heart failure.* Fall in EAV followed by salt and water retention and an increased venous return. Salt retention continues until the EAV is restored to the level necessary to excrete the daily salt load. The retained fluid expands the plasma volume and the ISF. If salt intake is restricted, a smaller EAV is required to excrete the salt load, and therefore less fluid is retained. In severe heart failure it becomes impossible to restore the EAV adequately, and salt retention continues with increasing oedema. Falling GFR results in renal tubular salt and water retention, and increasing venous pressure. As the cardiac output increases, pressure in the pulmonary capillaries increases, resulting in pleural effusion and increasing alveolar fluid, with symptoms of underperfusion.

2. In *potassium depletion* there is a tendency to the formation of mild oedema, with impaired heart muscle action. There is also impairment of the hyperaemic response to exercise in potassium-depleted muscles (? predisposes to rhabdomyolysis after prolonged exercise).

3. *Dialysis dysequilibrium syndrome.* Following rapid reduction of the urea concentration in the blood, late in the course of dialysis or several hours after completion, brain oedema develops—water drawn into the brain cells which still have a high urea concentration.

4. Toxaemia of pregnancy—there is salt retention, reduced GFR, rising blood pressure, increasing sensitivity to the action of angiotensin, with generalized oedema, including face and hands.

5. In normal pregnancy oedema of the feet and ankles is common at the end of the day in the third trimester. This oedema clears overnight at rest, and is due to high venous and capillary pressure in the legs due to increased venous capacitance and pressure of the gravid uterus on the inferior vena cava plus reduced plasma protein oncotic pressure.

6. During rapid fall of blood glucose during the treatment of diabetic keto acidosis water flows into the ICF, including the brain cells, and cerebral oedema may develop.

7. Heat oedema—increased salt and water retention (associated with salt supplements plus oliguria) causes oedema in unacclimatized people exposed to great heat.

8. Liver disease—(*a*) tense ascites exerting hydrostatic pressure and causing oedema in the lower limbs; (*b*) low plasma oncotic pressure due to low albumin concentration; (*c*) sodium retention and increased plasma volume.

9. In nephrosis, oedema occurs as the plasma albumin falls to low level, e.g. less than 20 g/l.

N.B. In primary salt retention which occurs in primary hyper-aldosteronism there is no oedema.

In primary water retention which occurs in inappropriate ADH secretion there is no oedema—the greater part of the fluid retention is in the ICF.

Treatment of Oedema

Treat the cause, whether local or general.

Restriction of daily salt intake—the normal daily salt intake comprises (150–200 mmol Na^+): 25 per cent occurring in the food; 25 per cent added during cooking; 50 per cent added at table (varying with habit)

Diuretics.

Salt-low albumin.

Care
  Hypotension ⎫
  Arrhythmias ⎬ if diuresis occurs.
  Hypokalaemia ⎭

Ascites—diuretics may reduce EAV, leading to hypotension and tubular necrosis, and encephalopathy.

Non-cardiac pulmonary oedema—'shock' lung requires urgent adequate oxygen plus treatment of the cause.

Pulmonary Oedema (Transudation of fluid into the pulmonary air spaces)

Acute Left Ventricular Failure

The pressure in lung capillaries lies between pulmonary artery pressure and left atrial pressure, at approximately 8 mmHg, which is lower than the equivalent pressure in the systemic circulation capillaries. The colloid osmotic pressure due to the plasma proteins is the same in both pulmonary and systemic circulations. When the capillary pressure in the lung reaches 30 mmHg, fluid enters the alveoli. The normal pulmonary ISF makes up 20 per cent of the lung mass, and cannot increase by more than 50 per cent before fluid escapes into the alveoli.

After an acute myocardial infarct, acute pulmonary oedema can develop within 15–20 min.

Acute Heart Failure Superimposed upon Chronic Heart Failure

Increasing pulmonary congestion results in reduced oxygenation of the blood, with increasing peripheral hypoxia. This causes peripheral vasodilatation. The increased venous return, following peripheral vasodilatation, causes increased pulmonary congestion, a vicious circle of deterioration developing.

Accumulation of fluid in the lungs increases tissue resistance, with expansion and contraction of the lungs during respiration becoming more difficult, and requiring increased work by the respiratory muscles. The normal lung tissue consumes about 4 per cent of the total body uptake of oxygen. Poorly oxygenated areas of lung develop increased permeability to fluid, so that patches of pulmonary oedema appear.

Chronic Left Ventricular Failure and Mitral Stenosis

There is protection from the development of pulmonary oedema by extremely rapid run-off of fluid from the pulmonary interstitial spaces into the lymphatics. When the pulmonary capillary pressure has been increased for 2 weeks, the pulmonary lymphatics enlarge 6–10 fold, and lymph flow increases twenty times the normal resting flow rate.

'Protective vasoconstriction' of the pulmonary arterioles has been postulated in chronic pulmonary venous hypertension with increased lymph flow.

Expansion of the ECF, with a sympathetic nervous system component, plus increased peripheral venous return, results in the pulmonary capillary pressure exceeding the plasma colloid osmotic pressure. When the capacity of the pulmonary lymphatics is exceeded, pulmonary oedema develops.

It is claimed that the pulmonary artery wedge pressure is normal, and that there is hypoxic vasoconstriction in the viscera. Leakage of fluid occurs in those regions of the pulmonary capillary bed not protected from high pulmonary artery pressure.

The force tending to keep the alveoli dry is equal to the difference between the osmotic pressure exerted by the plasma proteins and the capillary blood pressure, ignoring surface tension effects. In small alveoli the surface tension would tend to cause their collapse, but 'surfactant' in the lung alveoli reduces this tendency.

Damage of Local Capillary Membranes in the Lungs leading to pulmonary oedema:

1. Bacterial infection, e.g. pneumonia.
2. Irritant gases, e.g. chlorine, phosgene, smoke, etc.

Acute Decreases in Plasma Colloid Osmotic Pressure

Sudden massive infusion of non-colloid fluids.

Acute Increase in Pulmonary Capillary Pressure (Iatrogenic)

Gross transfusion overload with any infusion, including blood, plasma, saline, etc.

High Altitude Exposure

Pulmonary oedema occurs in some subjects, following rapid ascent to high altitude, accompanied by heavy physical activity. It is associated with marked pulmonary hypertension and normal left atrial pressure.

Onset of Pulmonary Oedema from any Cause

The development and severity of pulmonary oedema depends on:

1. The rate of change in pulmonary capillary pressure increase.
2. The rate of change in plasma colloid oncotic pressure.
3. The rate of development and severity of damage to the pulmonary capillary membranes.

Treatment of Acute Pulmonary Oedema

The patient is propped up and given morphine or an analogue, intravenous frusemide bolus (20–60 mg) and possibly aminophylline 0·25 g intravenously. Digoxin may also be given if indicated (e.g. mitral stenosis with fast atrial fibrillation). Hypertensive patients require antihypertensive therapy. Venous occlusion cuffs can be put on all four limbs, each cuff being deflated in rotation for 5 min every 15 min, or venesection may be undertaken, unless there is severe hypotension. Intermittent positive-pressure respiration may be useful, by reducing the venous return.

When pulmonary oedema follows inhalation of irritant gases, antibiotics and possibly steroids may be indicated.

In 'alveolar–capillary' block there is often hyperventilation with increased elimination of carbon dioxide and poor oxygenation, resulting in a low P_{CO_2} and a falling P_{O_2} (carbon dioxide being much more soluble and permeable than oxygen).

Brain Oedema

The brain weighs approximately 1400 g, with an 80 per cent water content (higher in the grey matter than the white matter). The brain blood volume is about 75 ml, with a flow rate of 750 ml/min. The intracranial cerebrospinal fluid has a volume of about 75 ml.

The normal intracranial pressure is less than 15 mmHg (measured in the lateral decubitus position), and shows pulsatile pressures synchronous with systole and diastole.

When intracranial pressure is abnormally increased (greater than 15 mmHg), plateau Lundberg waves occur in the presence of raised intracranial pressure plus brain oedema. These last for 5–20 min, before rapid return to interplateau pressure levels.

Increase in the volume of the brain is due to increase in its water content, and as brain oedema develops, water accumulates in the white matter and then in the grey matter, and herniation of the brain may occur.

Signs and Symptoms

Headache is severe, with vomiting. Papilloedema is seen. The patient becomes increasingly drowsy until consciousness is lost. There is loss of the ability to look upwards. Later, there is dilatation of the pupils, with loss of response to light. There is diffuse slowing of the EEG.

If intracranial pressure is high in the posterior fossa, then bradycardia and systemic hypertension develop.

Brain oedema is worsened by hypoxia, hypercapnoea and/or hyperthermia.

Clinical Varieties of Brain Oedema

1. *Vasogenic oedema*

The transport system of the choroid plexus removes organic acids, bases, ions and metabolites from the cerebrospinal fluid to the plasma, and hence from the brain ECF. With increased permeability of the brain capillary endothelial cells, brain tissue becomes oedematous, and the white matter is more vulnerable to this form of oedema than is the grey matter.

Causes

    a Brain tumour.
    b Brain abscess.
    c Brain haemorrhage.
    d Brain infarction.
    e Brain contusion.
    f Lead encephalopathy.
    g Purulent meningitis.

2. *Cytotoxic oedema*

All the cellular elements of the brain, including neurons, glia and endothelial cells, may swell, with reduction in the extracellular fluid spaces of the brain. The cells swell within seconds of hypoxia, because of failure of the cellular membrane ATP-ase dependent sodium pump. When the endothelial cells are particularly affected, the resistance to arterial perfusion of the brain is increasing, compounding existing hypoxia. Capillary permeability is usually not affected.

Causes

    a Hypoxia.
    b Acute hypo-osmolality.
        i Water intoxication
        ii SIADH.
        iii Acute sodium depletion.
    c Generalized brain oedema due to cerebral hypoxia, with hypercapnoea and severe acidosis.

Brain oedema does not occur in chronic hyponatraemia which has developed slowly.

Cerebral artery occlusion results in both vasogenic and cytotoxic brain oedema. High altitude cerebral oedema is thought to be hypoxic in origin.

3. *Interstitial oedema*

This form of brain oedema occurs in obstructive hydrocephalus. There is an increase in water and sodium content of periventricular white matter, due to movement of CSF across the ventricular walls.

In benign intracranial hypertension (pseudotumour cerebri) oedema is possibly due to defective absorption of cerebrospinal fluid at the arachnoid villi, resulting in a form of interstitial oedema.

4. Following rapid treatment of prolonged diabetic hyperglycaemia there is raised glucose concentration in the brain ISF and ICF, which lags behind the rapid fall in plasma glucose, and water is drawn into the brain cells. Normally brain glucose never exceeds 25 per cent of the plasma concentration. Insulin is associated with generation of 'idiogenic osmols'.
5. Dialysis disequilibrium syndrome: this occurs late in the course of renal haemodialysis, if dialysis is rapid. The normal gradient between blood and brain is 6 mmol/l, and urea may still be at higher concentration in the brain cells.

Treatment

1. Relieve any hypoxia (and obviously treat cardiac arrest).
2. Plasma hyperosmolality
If the blood–brain barrier is intact, various agents can be given to draw water from the brain back into the plasma, but this only occurs from normal brain tissue:
    a   Mannitol 20 per cent solution, 1–1·5 g/kg body weight is given intravenously over a period of 15–20 min. Some authorities also give frusemide.
    b   Urea 30 per cent solution in 10 per cent dextrose (1–1·5 g/kg body weight) is given intravenously to a maximum dose of 90 g. Unfortunately there may be late diffusion of urea into the brain, causing a dangerous rebound rise in brain tension.
3. Hyperventilation—this treats any hypoxia, and by producing hypocapnoea, also reduces intracranial pressure by reducing brain blood flow. The aim is to reduce the $Paco_2$ to 3·4–4·1 kPa (25–30 mmHg).
4. An alternative to hyperventilation is hyperbaric oxygen, which has also been used when facilities are available.
5. Controlled hypotension and hypothermia. Hyperthermia is dangerous in brain oedema.
6. Steroids—dexamethasone 10 mg stat, followed by 4 mg 6-hourly for 2–3 days has been found to reduce brain oedema, especially if caused by cerebral tumour or abscess. There is a serious risk of gastric haemorrhages when such large doses are used, but steroid psychosis is only rarely seen.
7. Barbiturates—these have been used (e.g. pentobarbitone) in doses near to the level of toxicity, and while barbiturates do cause hypothermia, their value is questioned.
8. Althesin—This mixture of two anaesthetic steroids has given promising results in the treatment of brain oedema.
9. Surgery
    a   Surgical shunting is used in the treatment of interstitial

oedema due to obstructive hydrocephalus. Acetazolamide, which reduces the rate of production of cerebrospinal fluid, is only of limited value.
b   Surgical treatment of cerebral tumour or abscess.

Paracetamol (Acetaminophen) Poisoning
Molecular Weight
151.

Absorption
Rapid with peak at 1–3 h after dose.

Metabolism
1   Therapeutic dose
    a   Small fraction forms active metabolite binding with glutathione, and excreted as mercapturic acid. Rapidly inactivated.
    b   Most of remainder excreted as conjugates of glucuronide and sulphate, both pharmacologically inactive. Conjugative capacity exceeded by doses greater than 5 g, with damage to heart, liver, kidneys.
2   Toxic dose
    More active metabolite formed. If it is in excess of available cellular glutathione, it combines covalently with proteins in the cell cytosol and endoplasmic reticulum in the centrilobular zone, resulting in centrilobular necrosis. Phenobarbitone enhances hepatotoxicity. Available glutathione protects against cell necrosis.
    Hepatic glutathione is depleted by: diethyl maleate; fasting. Susceptibility increased by alcohol.
    Hepatic necrosis occurs when dose is large enough to deplete more than 70 per cent of the hepatic glutathione. Hepatic damage from dose exceeding 15 g may be fatal unless prompt correct treatment.

Biological Half-life
Usual pharmacological dose—2–3 h.
Large dose—4–5 h.
Combined with other drugs—4–5 h.
Five per cent of the dose is excreted unchanged in the urine.

Clinical Findings in Poisoning

Phase 1. Acute gastrointestinal symptoms—anorexia, nausea, vomiting.

Phase 2. Relative well-being without anorexia or vomiting, lasting for approx. 2 days. Usually oliguria.

Phase 3. Overt jaundice appears by third to fifth day, fulminant hepatic failure.

Haemorrhages, encephalopathy, death.

Toxicity correlates with blood levels:

More than 2 mmol (300 mg/100 ml) at 4 h—overt hepatic damage.

Less than 1 mmol (150 mg/100 ml) at 4 h—usually no hepatic damage.

Laboratory Test Results

Plot 2 mmol/l (200 mg/100 ml) at 4 h and 0·2 mmol/l (30 mg/100 ml) at 15 h on semilog. paper 0·4 mmol/l (60 mg/100 ml at 10 h) against time. Above the line = risk of damage, and need for active treatment.

High risk = more than 2 mmol/l (300 mg/100 ml) at 4 h, and above, 0·3 mmol/l (45 mg/100 ml) at 15 h.

Aspartate transaminase and alanine transaminase increased in proportion to cell necrosis in liver.

BCR (prothrombin ratio) increased above 2·0 = bad prognosis.

Disseminated intravascular coagulation (DIC) may develop late.

Treatment

Mercaptamine, methionine, cysteine, acetylcysteine all increase hepatic glutathione. Treatment with acetyl cysteine, or methionine, 'must' be within the first 12 hours (24 h at latest).

1   Methionine—2·5 g orally, with 2·5 g every 4 h depending on blood levels. *But* severely poisoned patient may suffer from nausea and vomiting.

2   Intravenous acetyl cysteine
     a   150 mg/kg in 200 ml 5 per cent dextrose over 15 min.
     b   50 mg/kg in 500 ml 5 per cent glucose over 4 h.
     c   50 mg/kg in 500 ml 5 per cent dextrose over 8 h.
     d   50 mg/kg in 500 ml 5 per cent dextrose over 8 h.

Acetylcysteine is associated with falling plasma potassium and falling bicarbonate, and sometimes thrombocytopenia in first 72 hours of treatment.

Renal Failure

Acute Renal Tubular Necrosis

The development of uraemic symptoms depends on the rate of tissue

catabolism in the patient with renal failure, which depends on:
1. Presence or absence of infection.
2. Amount of tissue trauma present.
3. Age and muscle mass of the patient.
4. Efficacy of any measures taken to reduce endogenous protein catabolism. In the early stages of acute tubular necrosis there is progressive reduction in urine flow over 24–48 h from the initial damage, falling to less than 50 ml of urine per day. This early urine will contain epithelial cells, epithelial cell casts and coarsely granular casts in most patients.

Non-oliguric acute tubular necrosis can occur, with no reduction in urine flow, in 30–60 per cent of cases. This may reflect the more frequent use of prophylactic mannitol infusons, 'loop' diuretics, and vasodilators in high-risk cases (very severe trauma, surgery and severe burns cases).

Acute tubular necrosis can be superimposed on chronic renal insufficiency, for example, aminoglycoside renal toxicity during treatment of infection with gentamicin.

During the first few days of oliguria the plasma concentration of urea, creatinine and uric acid increases, and metabolic acidosis develops because of the failure to excrete hydrogen ions. Plasma bicarbonate and pH fall with secondary relatively smaller decrease in Pa_{CO_2} (secondary compensation). If there is excess water in the body, hyponatraemia is found, with raised plasma magnesium, phosphate, and potassium from cells. Comparison of plasma and urine concentration ratios of urea, creatinine and osmolality show a progressive fall, as the ability of the kidney to concentrate urine disappears. Similarly, urine sodium concentration rises and exceeds 40 mmol/l (i.e. approaching plasma concentration).

With the increase in plasma inorganic phosphate, serum calcium levels may fall, but not to the same degree as in chronic renal failure.

After the initial phase of renal tubular necrosis there may be a stage when about 400 ml of urine are excreted each day, but the GFR is abnormally low, and excretion of solute is insufficient. When the patient has accumulated a water overload during the initial oliguric phase, massive diuresis of weak urine may occur, as the overload is corrected.

Urine concentrating ability remains defective for several months, but a period of rapid improvement in renal function may result in a late diuresis with blood urea concentration falling to normal. Maximum recovery of renal function may take up to a year to be complete.

Treatment

Prevention, if possible:
1 Maintenance of optimal tissue perfusion.

2 Mannitol infusion (500 ml of 20 per cent mannitol) over 24 h, if urine flow is maintained. Alternatively, 50 ml of 25 per cent mannitol solution can be given intravenously over 5–10 min, the dose repeated after 1 h if urine flow is increased but not maintained, no more mannitol being given if there is no change in urine flow. Excess infusion of mannitol results in fluid overload and pulmonary oedema with hyponatraemia, if kidney function is greatly impaired. The response to mannitol may be:

a No significant increase in the output of urine, when complete acute renal failure is present. No further fluid should be given until very careful clinical assessment has been made, because of the danger of fluid overload.

b Immediate and marked increase in urine output will suggest that there was prerenal azotaemia with resumption of normal renal function following mannitol infusion.

c There may be partial renal failure with increased urinary output, but creatinine clearance values remain low. 'Loop' diuretics should probably not be given to such oliguric patients, when acute tubular necrosis is suspected, but they may have a role in prevention, if given before potentially dangerous surgery is carried out.

Chronic Renal Failure with Uraemia
Signs and Symptoms

1. Gradually increasing polyuria and nocturia, with loss of the normal diurnal variation in urinary flow occurs, with the progressive reduction in the GFR and loss of concentration and dilution of urine.

When the GFR falls below 25 ml/min there is defective ammonia synthesis, ammonium production, and adequate hydrogen ion excretion. Metabolic acidosis develops. When this acidosis is severe, with low plasma bicarbonate concentration, low plasma pH and falling Pa_{CO_2}, respiration becomes slow and deep ('Kussmaul' respiration).

2. Patients suffer from nausea and diarrhoea, with bleeding into the gastrointestinal tract. Anaemia, with bleeding tendency due to impairment of platelet function by retained metabolites, occurs.

3. Congestive cardiac failure, high blood pressure and, later, pericarditis are found.

4. There is fat wasting, weakness and osteodystrophy, with falling plasma calcium, increasing plasma inorganic phosphate and secondary hyperparathyroidism.

5. When the GFR falls below 15–20 per cent of normal, homeostasis is difficult, the patient easily becoming dehydrated or overloaded with fluid, and with metabolites accumulating. Plasma magnesium, inorganic phosphate and potassium derived from cell breakdown and

metabolism, are not excreted adequately. Plasma urea, creatinine and uric acid concentrations increase progressively. The kidney's ability to concentrate or dilute urine is lost progressively.
6. With the loss of renal tissue, synthesis of $1,25-(OH)_2D_3$ falls, depressing calcium absorption from the gastrointestinal tract.
7. Sleep disturbance and personality changes which may progress to psychosis are found. The EEG readings are abnormal, and later convulsions occur.

Renal Tubular Acidosis Type I (Distal Gradient RTA)

The distal renal tubule is not able to initiate or maintain the normal pH difference between the plasma and the tubular urine, and the minimum urinary pH rises. Titratable acid falls and may be absent from the urine. The urine is inappropriately alkaline for the corresponding plasma pH, and does not fall below 6·0. Ammonia secretion by the tubules is normal or low, and there is a persistent hyperchloraemic acidosis without renal failure. The inability to excrete an acid urine can be demonstrated by an oral ammonium chloride load, 100 mg/kg orally should cause urine pH to fall below 5·5 during the next 5–6 h.

Causes

1 Idiopathic sporadic.
2 Mendelian dominant inheritance.
3 Secondary to:
    a Renal tract obstruction.
    b Pyelonephritis.
    c Hypercalcaemia, including primary hyperparathyroidism with nephrosclerosis.
    d Hepatic cirrhosis.
    e Mercury intoxication.
    f Medullary sponge kidney.
    g Following renal transplant.
    h Hypergammaglobulinaemia in autoimmune disease.
    i Amphotericin B intoxication.
    j Galactosaemia.
    k Hereditary fructose intolerance with nephrosclerosis.
    l Fabry's disease.
    m Ehlers–Danlos syndrome.

Complications

1 Renal sodium and potassium wastage.

2 Failing renal power to concentrate urine.
3 Medullary nephrocalcinosis.
4 Renal stone formation.
5 Renal rickets and osteomalacia.
6 Severe muscle weakness due to potassium wastage.

In the absence of treatment, metabolic acidosis persists and hypo-kalaemia may be severe. There is a risk of nephrolithiasis and nephrosclerosis. Because of the inability to generate bicarbonate in the distal tubules, hyperaldosteronism develops following sodium loss. With potassium loss and chloride retention, a hyperchloraemic acidosis develops. Secondary hyperparathyroidism follows the transient fall in plasma calcium, with hypercalciuria. Hypercalciuria in an alkaline urine results in nephrolithiasis and nephrocalcinosis.

Treatment

Sodium bicarbonate, 1–3 mmol/kg body weight are given each day, with potassium supplements if plasma potassium is low.

Renal Tubular Acidosis Type 2 (Proximal, Rate RTA)

There is reduced ability of the renal proximal tubules to produce a normal rate of tubular hydrogen ion secretion, resulting in loss of an appreciable amount of bicarbonate in the urine. A persistent hyper-chloraemic acidosis develops which is very resistant to treatment with alkalis, and the urine pH falls to very low levels.

Following a bicarbonate load orally, plasma bicarbonate concentration does not return to normal levels, and potassium wasting persists. With the bicarbonate load, the urine pH rises to 5·5–6·0.

Causes

1 Primary
    a Infantile
        i Transient.
        ii Persistent.
    b Sporadic.
    c Genetic.
2 Secondary
    a Secondary hyperparathyroidism.
    b Intoxication with degraded tetracyclines.
    c Following renal transplant.
    d Heavy metal intoxication.
    e Medullary cystic disease.
    f Nephrotic syndrome.

g Sjögren's syndrome.
h Galactosaemia.
i Wilson's hepatolenticular disease.
j Multiple myelomatosis.
k Amyloidosis.
l Cystinosis.
m Familial fructose intolerance.

Complications

1 Potassium depletion.
2 Rickets.
3 Nephrocalcinosis is rare.
Affecting more females than males.

Onset

1 In infants without other renal lesions.
2 In adults with amino-aciduria, glycosuria or hypophosphataemia (Fanconi syndrome).

Treatment

Treatment is not satisfactory, although severe cases may benefit from a low salt diet with thiazide diuretics. In adults the condition is usually mild.

Renal Tubular Acidosis Type 4

There is impaired renal acidification with reduced renal clearance of potassium. This results in plasma hyperkalaemia, with metabolic acidosis, hyporeninaemia and hypoaldosteronism. The urine ammonium excretion rate is reduced even though the urine is acid.

Causes

1 Aldosterone deficiency
   a Adrenal hypocorticalism (Addison's disease).
   b Post-bilateral adrenalectomy.
   c Congenital adrenal hyperplasia.
2 Selective deficiency of aldosterone
   a Inherited corticosterone methyloxidase deficiency.
   b Secondary to renin secretion deficiency.
   c Chronic idiopathic hypoaldosteronism.

3   Attenuated renal response to aldosterone
    a Selective renal tubular dysfunction—pseudohypoaldosteron-
         ism.
    b Chronic interstitial and tubular disease with glomerular insuf-
         ficiency ('salt wasting').
4   Attenuated renal response to aldosterone and aldosterone
    deficiency
    a Selective tubular dysfunction and impaired renin secretion.
    b Chronic tubulo-interstitial deficiency with glomerular
         insufficiency.
    c Deficient renin secretion—postrenal transplant; systemic lupus
         erythematosus.
5   Others
    a Acute glomerulonephritis.
    b Chronic pyelonephritis.
    c Lupus nephritis.
    d Post-renal transplant.

Treatment

1   9-α-Fluorocortisone (fludrocortisone) 0·1–0·3 mg daily.
2   Restrict loop diuretics.
3   Restrict dietary potassium (i.e. avoid potassium-rich foods where
possible).
4   Sodium bicarbonate 1·5–2 mmol/kg/day.
5   Some children respond to chlorothiazide diuretic.

Salicylate Poisoning
Molecular Weight

1   Aspirin = 180.
2   Sodium salicylate = 160.
3   Salicylic acid = 138 (the active principle in the circulation).

Absorption
Rapid.

Biological Half-life
Aspirin (acetylsalicylic acid) = 15 min only.
Acetylsalicylic acid 300 mg (as salicylic acid) = 2–3 h.
    Therapeutic dose (as salicylic acid) = 6–12 h.
    Toxic doses (as salicylic acid) = 20 h +.

Metabolism

Acetylsalicyclic acid is converted to salicylic acid during and after absorption. Of the salicylic acid 70–90 per cent is bound to plasma protein.

Conjugation:
1 Some salicylic acid is conjugated with glycine to form salicyluric acid.
2 Some salicylic acid is excreted as acyl glucuronide.
3 Some salicylic acid is excreted as phenyl glucuronide.
4 Some salcylic acid is hydroxylated to gentisic acid, which is metabolically active.
There is limited capacity for the salicylic acid and salicylyl-phenolic glucuronide pathways.

Excretion

Less than 10 per cent excreted unchanged in the urine on low dosage. More than 50 per cent is excreted unchanged in the urine on high dosage. Any renal dysfunction slows excretion after large dosage. Unless there is circulatory collapse, 50 per cent of the ingested salicylate is excreted during the first 24 hours in alkaline urine, during forced alkaline diuresis.

Toxicity

1 Doses less than 150 mg/kg = negligible effects.
2 Doses exceeding 500 mg/kg = potentially lethal (e.g. adult ingesting 25–30 g).

Clinical Signs and Symptoms

When plasma levels exceed 2·9 mmol/l (40 mg/dl) the patient suffers from tinnitus. At higher blood levels there is peripheral vasodilatation, sweating, hyperpnoea and hyperthermia. Abdominal pain may be accompanied by vomiting. By preventing rouleaux formation, the ESR is normal. Later, hypothermia develops with pulmonary oedema and hypoglycaemia (with fatty liver). Twitching may progress to frank convulsions. Plasma potassium levels fall. There may be spontaneous bleeding. Electroencephalograph readings are abnormal, and hallucinations may occur ('salicylate jag').

Active treatment should be instituted if plasma salicylate exceeds 0·36 mmol/l (50 mg/dl) in adults, or 0·22 mmol/l (30 mg/dl) in children.

Clinicopathology

There is salicylate-induced uncoupling of normal oxidative phosphorylation which results in increased carbon dioxide production, and an increase up to +40 per cent of the basal metabolic rate, with increased depth, and then rate, of respiration.

Stimulation of the respiratory centre in the medulla causes respiratory alkalosis, when the plasma salicylate level reaches 2·9 mmol/l. Later, the medulla is depressed, when pulmonary oedema develops, and respiratory acidosis occurs.

Salicylate dissociates in the plasma, releasing free hydrogen ions, and causing metabolic acidosis due to a non-volatile organic acid. Pyruvate and lactate concentrations increase in the plasma and the ECF. There is inhibition of Krebs cycle enzymes and inhibition of amino-acid metabolism.

The low $P\text{aco}_2$ associated with respiratory alkalosis, results in increased loss of sodium, potassium and water in the urine. Sodium and potassium transport across cell membranes is inhibited, with loss of potassium from cells and entry of sodium and hydrogen ions into the cells.

Renal glucose reabsorption from the glomerular filtrate is reduced, the liver glycogen stores are rapidly depleted, and fatty infiltration of the liver may develop, with impairment of glucose metabolism. Infants can develop very serious hypoglycaemia. The fatal dose of aspirin is thought to be about 10–30 g, although up to 130 g have been ingested by some suicides, and the recent development of slow-release enteric coated salicylate capsules means that after an overdose with such tablets, there may be prolonged continuous release and hence absorption of salicylate.

Treatment

Salicylate moves in undissociated form from one tissue compartment to another. During forced alkaline diuresis, salicylate is eliminated, but excretion is incomplete during diuretic therapy until the urine is alkaline. Five hundred ml 1·4 per cent sodium bicarbonate

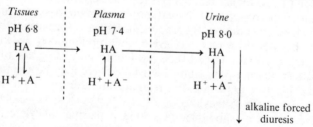

HA represents the undissociated salicylate.

(167 mmol/l), 500 ml 5 per cent dextrose solution and 500 ml 0·9 per cent sodium chloride (15 mmol/l) are given in rotation at the rate of 2 litres per hour (if urine flow is satisfactory). Once diuresis has started, potassium chloride supplements should be added at the rate of 15 mmol per 500 ml of fluid, after the first hour, when urine flow is good. Potassium supplements are needed, since alkalinization of the urine is incomplete in the presence of uncorrected potassium depletion. Potassium supplements can be reduced or discontinued, once the urine pH is alkaline.

Laboratory Findings after Toxic Doses

Combination of respiratory alkalosis, metabolic acidosis plus dehydration.

AST × 10 above normal.
ALT × 10 above normal.
Bilirubin in serum slight increase.
BCR (prothrombin ratio) × 2.

Blood Salicylate Levels

	6 hours	24 hours	36 hours
Asymptomatic	0·33 mmol/l (<45 mg/dl)	0·18 mmol/l (<25 mg/dl)	0·11 mmol/l (<15 mg/dl)
Moderate	0·47–0·65 mmol/l (65–90 mg/dl)	0·29–0·4 mmol/l (40–55 mg/dl)	0·18–0·24 mmol/l (25–33 mg/dl)
Severe	0·87 mmol/dl (>120 mg/dl)	0·54 mmol/l (>75 mg/dl)	0·33 mmol/l (>45 mg/dl)

Shock

Ten per cent of the total blood volume can be lost fairly rapidly without marked symptoms, e.g normal blood donor. The blood lost is rapidly replaced by diffusion from the ISF resulting in a lower whole blood haemoglobin on the next day (e.g. 15 g/dl falls to 13·5 g/dl overnight). The haemoglobin and red cells are replaced during the next few weeks—the rate of haematopoiesis is directly proportional to the depression of the haemoglobin concentration.

Haemorrhagic shock develops when 25–30 per cent of the total blood volume is lost fairly rapidly, i.e. over a period of minutes to hours, with a loss of about 1500 ml of blood. Shock in this situation is due to generalized tissue anoxia and the body's response to the anoxia. The circulation readjusts to maintain a priority blood supply to the brain and the heart, reducing blood flow to:

1 Kidneys—with blood flow diverted from cortical nephrons to the long-loop juxtamedullary nephrons.

2 Lungs (with shunting).

3 Gastrointestinal tract.
4 Peripheral circulation.
The severity of signs and symptoms are directly related to the rate of blood loss.
Other varieties of shock include:
1 Cardiogenic shock.
2 Hypovolaemic shock.
3 Vasomotor shock.

Signs and Symptoms

Include:

Apprehension.   Pallor.
Weakness.   Tachycardia.
Cold extremities.   Loss of consciousness.
Low blood pressure.

Generalized vasodilatation develops in irreversible shock, the so-called 'shock-begetting-shock' in which it has been thought the 'sick cell syndrome' develops—with the failure of the cell membrane sodium pump, and sodium, water and hydrogen ions entering cells and loss of intracellular potassium. The existence of the 'sick cell syndrome' is debated, but if it exists, it must have far-reaching consequences, since the sodium pump is fundamental to renal function. With low blood pressure, oliguria develops. If the renal perfusing pressure falls below 70–80 mmHg (systolic), urine flow ceases. Urine flow ceases when there is a 20 per cent deficit in the circulating blood volume. (The normal urine flow averages 1 ml/kg body weight/h.)

In man there is increasing congestion in the lungs with shunting of the blood flow, i.e. blood passes more rapidly through the lungs without being properly oxygenated. Stress ulcers may develop in the stomach, and disseminated intravascular coagulopathy may develop (especially in association with Gram-negative bacterial septicaemia). Blood lactate and blood glucose concentrations may rise, with a falling plasma pH (increasing hydrogen ion concentration).

Central Venous Pressure

The normal central venous pressure is about 10 mmHg (with a normal upper limit of 15 mmHg). It falls towards zero in increasingly severe haemorrhagic shock due to blood loss. If it rises towards 20 mmHg, it heralds the onset of pulmonary oedema, indicating the failure of the right ventricle to move blood from the lungs.

Sick Cell Syndrome

After injury, major surgery, burns in the first few days, severe myocardial infarction, severe congestive cardiac failure, and other severe illnesses, including gram-negative septicaemia, hyponatraemia with large losses of potassium in the urine may occur. It has been postulated that the sick cell syndrome involves a loss of integrity of the cell membranes, and originally it was suggested that potassium (with magnesium and phosphate) left the cells to be replaced by sodium and hydrogen ions. No such gross movement of sodium into cells has been found. It has also been suggested that the high-pressure and low-pressure baroreceptors and osmoreceptors may be responding to apparently contradictory stimuli (e.g. falling circulatory effective volume versus increased pulmonary pressure). More probably, non-diffusible, predominantly anionic solutes normally held inside cells escape into the ECF through leaky cell membranes. The fall in intracellular osmolality is then balanced by a fall in ECF osmolality with reduction in plasma sodium concentration.

Responses to hypovolaemia, or apparent hypovolaemia, with reduced ECV override responses to changes in osmolality detected by osmoreceptors. There can be different responses from high-pressure baroreceptors and low-pressure baroreceptors when cardiac failure is predominantly right-sided or left-sided.

The apparent satisfactory clinical response to the treatment of the sick cell syndrome, namely intravenous glucose (50 g i.v.) and insulin 20 u i.v. three to four times daily, followed by adequate feeding (and many of the clinical conditions associated with sick cell syndrome are hypercatabolic), with return of the plasma sodium towards normal and the urine potassium output falling, with increased sodium excretion in the urine, could reflect satisfactory adjustment of intracellular anion, cation and water plus nutrition, combined with consequent adjustment of the ECF. More readily available direct osmolality measurements will help to define and analyse this condition in the future.

Starvation

Normal calorie intake is approximately 2500 calories per day.
During starvation with unrestricted fluid available:

Body glycogen (400–600 g) rapidly used up (exhausted within a few hours of the last meal).

Body fat catabolized for energy. One g releases 9 calories plus 1 ml water (with no release of sodium chloride).

Muscle protein catabolized for: release of amino acids and carbohydrates for gluconeogenesis.

One g muscle releases 1 calorie plus potassium and nitrogen and water (with no release of sodium chloride). (Muscle is the main body reserve for protein and also potassium.)

Body weight loss = 300 g/day at least. At the end of 3 weeks without adequate intake 15 per cent of body weight is lost.

The basal metabolic rate falls, and the CNS adapts to oxidation of ketones (plus glucose) which reduces gluconeogenesis and spares protein. There is a high mortality rate after 40 per cent loss of body weight.

USEFUL SOLUTIONS; USEFUL FORMULAE

Solutions

	Sodium	Potassium	Calcium	Chloride	Bicarbonate	Lactate	Ammonium	Phosphate
					mmol/litre			
0·18% Sodium chloride	31			31				
0·3% Sodium chloride	51			51				
0·45% Sodium chloride	77			77				
0·9% Sodium chloride	150			150				
1·8% Sodium chloride	308			308				
1·4% Sodium bicarbonate	167				167			
2·74% Sodium bicarbonate	326				326			
4·2% Sodium bicarbonate	500				500			
8·4% Sodium bicarbonate	1000				1000			
0·3% Potassium chloride		40		40				
M/6 Sodium lactate	167					167		
M/6 (0·5%) Ammonium chloride				167			167	
Sodium potassium phosphate	162	19						100
Hartman	131	5	2	111		29		
Ringer	147	4	2	155				
Darrow	121	35		103		53		

	Sodium	Potassium	mmol/ampoule Calcium	Chloride	Magnesium	Phosphate
Ampoules containing per ampoule						
Calcium chloride			10			
Calcium gluconate			2·23			
Potassium chloride						
1 g in 10 ml		13				
1·5 g in 10 ml		20				
2 g in 10 ml		26				
50% Magnesium chloride (2 ml)					4	
17·42% Potassium phosphate 10 ml						10

Dextrose	*Dextrose (g/l)*	*Dextrose (mmol/l)*	*Dextrose (calories)*
5%	50	278	205
10%	100	556	410
20%	200	1112	820

Formulae
Calculations and Approximations and Definitions

Total Carbon Dioxide Concentration

Total carbon dioxide extractable from plasma in the presence of a strong acid. Represents the total dissolved carbon dioxide, carbonic acid, bicarbonate ion, carbonate ion and carbamino compounds. This estimation should be used when anion gap is considered.

Plasma Bicarbonate Ion Concentration

Concentration of bicarbonate in plasma = total carbon dioxide minus dissolved carbon dioxide (+carbamino compounds).

Standard Bicarbonate Concentration

The concentration of bicarbonate in plasma of oxygenated whole blood which has been equilibrated to a P_{CO_2} of 40 mmHg at 37 °C before separation of plasma.

Buffer Base

The sum of the concentration of buffer anions in whole blood. The normal buffer base = the normal buffer base for the particular haemoglobin concentration of the blood sample.

Base Excess

Base concentration of whole blood measured by titration with strong acid to bring the plasma pH to 7·40 at a P_{CO_2} of 3 kPa (40 mmHg) at 37 °C. Base deficit—for negative values, titration is with strong base. (Using the Siggaard–Andersen nomogram system—the line passing through the observed P_{CO_2} and pH reads off base excess according to haemoglobin concentration, and give the actual plasma bicarbonate concentration. The line passing through the base excess reading to a P_{CO_2} reading to 40 mmHg reads back to the standard bicarbonate.)

Sodium Deficit

In hypotonic dehydration, following loss of ECF and partial fluid replacement, with weight loss (i.e. not overhydration),

Sodium deficit = (140 − Patient's plasma sodium) × total body water (litres)

e.g. = (140 − 120) × Body Wt (kg) × 0·5 mmol sodium deficit.

Water Excess

In hypotonic overhydration, with hyponatraemia and weight gain,

$$\text{Water excess} = \text{Body wt (kg)} \times 0.6 \left(1 - \frac{\text{Patient's Na}}{140\,\text{mmol/l}}\right) \text{ litres of water.}$$

Water Deficit

In hypernatraemic dehydration, with weight loss,

1. $\text{Water deficit} = \dfrac{\text{Body wt (kg)}}{2} \left(1 - \dfrac{140\,\text{mmol/l}}{\text{Patient's Na}}\right)$ litres of water,

or

2. $\dfrac{\text{Body weight (lb)}}{100}\ \dfrac{(\text{Patient's Na} - 140\,\text{mmol/l})}{6}$ litres of water,

or

3. $\dfrac{\text{Body weight (kg)}}{100}\ \dfrac{\text{Patient's Na} - 140}{13.2}$ litres of water.

Plasma Osmolality (approximately)

$= 2 \times \text{plasma sodium (mmol/l)} + \text{glucose (mmol/l)} + \text{urea (mmol/l)}$
$= \text{approx. } 295\,\text{mmosmol/kg.}$

It is important to note when this calculated osmolality is significantly different from the observed measurement of plasma osmolality.

Bicarbonate Deficit

Normal plasma bicarbonate is approximately 24 mmol/l.

$$(24 - \text{patient's bicarbonate}) \times \frac{\text{Patient's wt (kg)}}{5} = \text{ECF bicarbonate}$$

deficit in mmol.

The total deficit is probably four times this calculation, but correction should only be to the ECF value first. Any change in bicarbonate during therapy results in continuous adjustment of plasma pH and CO_2. Careful empirical therapy is more sensible.

Base Excess

Negative Base excess $\times 0.3 \times$ kg body weight
= mmol deficit in ECF as sodium bicarbonate.

Positive base excess $\times 0.3 \times$ kg body weight
= mmol ammonium chloride to bring pH in alkalosis back to normal.

INDEX

Passim means 'here and there throughout'.